EXTREME BRAIN REANIMATION

THE FRANKENSTEIN EFFECT

Prof. Sergio Canavero, MD

DISCLAIMER: This is a technical book for medical professionals. It is not intended for use by lay persons. The author assumes no responsibility for any improper use of the contents thereof.

By far the greatest obstacle to the progress of science...is...that men...think things impossible

Francis Bacon

Convey an energetic fluid to the seat of all sensations; distribute its force throughout the different parts of the nervous and muscular systems; produce, reanimate and, so to speak, control the vital forces: this is the object of my research

Giovanni Aldini

Discovery consists of seeing what everybody has seen and thinking what nobody has thought

Albert Szent-Gyorgy

ΔΑΙΜΩΝ   ΗΘΟϹ

CONTENTS

PREFACE

Upon a slight conjecture I have ventured on a dangerous journey,
   And I already behold the foothills of new lands -
   Those who have the courage to continue the search
will set foot upon them.

Immanuel Kant

My involvement with the science described in this book began in the 1990's, when my life-long focus on the nature of consciousness had peaked. At the time, I was experimenting with electrical cortical stimulation of the brain for relief of pain and movement disorders (reviewed in **Canavero 2009, 2014**), but my fixation was with the so-called Permanent Vegetative States, in which the patient is apparently unaware of the world around as a result of global brain ischemia that lasts too long. By my lights, this condition could have advanced our meager understanding of conscious processes. After many (despairing) years, finally I got the chance to stimulate the cortex of two such young subjects in 2007: to my disbelief, what was considered irreversible, turned out not to be, as –for the first time ever- both moved up a step in the consciousness continuum to minimally conscious (**Canavero et al 2009**). Project Lazarus (as I named it: **Canavero 2010**) was ambitious: stimulation should have been boosted by the intrathecal infusion of mesenchymal stem cells (something that proved impossible to do in Italy). This early (very partial) success galvanized me and led me to rethink all that I had been taught. I ventured further...

The question I will tackle in this book is thus straightforward: can a previously healthy human – say, a competitive athlete- who has been pronounced dead because of global brain ischemia following sudden, irreversible cardiac death be brought back to life several hours later fully sentient and cognitively intact?

According to medical lore, the answer is an unqualified

NO!

According to this lore, mammalian brains, in light of their voracious energy demands, are highly susceptible to anoxia and glucose deprivation (as occurs -for instance- with cessation of blood flow, a.k.a. ischemia). Studies in both humans and experimental animals have shown that this deprivation causes loss of consciousness in approximately 5–7 seconds followed by the electroencephalogram (EEG) going flat within 15–20 seconds. Anerobic glycolysis can support a maximum of 1-2 minutes of normal metabolism. Unless perfusion is quickly restored, multiple deleterious mechanisms lead to widespread membrane depolarization, loss of ionic homeostasis, mitochondrial dysfunction, and excitotoxic accumulation of glutamate and consequently cell death within 4-6 minutes (**Safar 1996**).

In this book, I beg to differ, as I set out to explore the rationale that subtends what in a paper published in 2016 I named the **Frankenstein Effect (Canavero et al 2016)**: resuscitation of the brain **at least 6** hours after "death". Damaged organs can be replaced, a hugely damaged body can be replaced (one day even with a cloned body) (**Canavero 2013, 2014a**). But the brain is the pivotal organ that filters consciousness into everyone's individuality (**Canavero 2014b**).

To achieve this goal, we must ask ourselves: When does life end?

Presently, there is no consensus on a definition of "life". In this book, we will thus make an assumption :

Life becomes impossible ONLY after complete cellular dissolution.

Partial damage and/or even severe dysfunction is not equivalent to irreversible loss of that cell or its function, even if that cell is metabolically and electrophysiologically silent.

We will thus endeavor to establish temporal limits for any extreme brain reanimation (EBR)- "Frankenstein Effect" (FE) protocols (EBR-FE) and possible ways to restart normal cellular function and all those processes that allow the brain to filter consciousness (**NOTE 1**).

CHAPTER 1

JOLTING THE DEAD

ACADEMY OF SCIENCES, TURIN, NORTHERN ITALY,
THE 27ᵀᴴ DAY OF THERMIDOR, YEAR 10
(AUGUST 15, 1802)

A demonstration is being held held on the effects of galvanism applied to human cadavers. In particular, the method developed by Prof. Giovanni Aldini from Bologna is being tested on three decapitated convicts.

"Le Comité de Turin décrit l'étonnement dont furent frappés les spectateurs de leurs expériences galvaniques, en voyant dans le cadavre de l'homme les contractions des muscles...de la face...de la langue...du dos, qui élevaient le tronc de quelques pouces sur la table...Les contractions du bras...étaient tellement promptes et violentes, que l'entière flexion de l'avant-bras sur le bras avait lieu, et que le main enlevait un poids de quelques livres plus de 50 minutes après de la

*décapitation...Les muscles du bras, du dos et de la poitrine, continuent a être excitables par le galvanisme **des heures entières**...le cœur avait perdu son excitabilité dès la quarantième minute environ après la mort...* » **(Aldini 1803).**

*["The Turin Committee describes the astonishment of the spectators for their galvanic experiences, seeing in the corpse of the man the contractions of the muscles ... of the face ... of the tongue ... of the back, which raised the trunk by a few inches off the table ... The contractions of the arm ... were so quick and violent, that the forearm fully flexed on the arm, and the hand lifted a weight of a few pounds more than 50 minutes after the decapitation ... The muscles of the arm, back and chest, continue to be excitable by galvanism **for hours** ... the heart had lost its excitability in the fortieth minute after death..."]*

?

Between the end of the XVIII century and the start of the XIX century, at the height of the controversy on the existence of animal electricity between Alessandro Volta (con) and Luigi Galvani (pro), Giovanni Aldini, Galvani's nephew, in order to prove his uncle right, applied electrical stimulation ("galvanism") first to animals, then to humans. Employing Volta's battery ("Pila") in Bologna (Northern Italy), he produced all manner of muscular contractions by applying an electric arc at different points along the head and bodies. He then stimulated various regions of the human brain: **massive facial muscle contractions were generated by stimulating the callosal fibers and the cerebral cortex**.

In January 1803, Aldini conducted an experiment in London on George Foster who had been hanged and left in the cold for 1 hour. The movements induced were *"so much increased as almost to give the appearance of reanimation."* The news was reported by The Times on January 22, 1803, and strongly and enduringly impressed scientists and ordinary people alike, many coming to believe that electricity might be the long-sought vital force. This belief later inspired Mary Shelley and her novel Frankenstein in 1818.

In 1804, Aldini reported on further experiments on a decapitated body: the body became violently agitated and even raised itself as if about to walk, the arms alternately rose and fell and the forearm was made to hold a weight of several pounds , while the fists clenched and beat violently the table upon which the body lay. Natural respiration was also artificially reestablished.

Many other physicians later replicated Aldini's results (see **Mottelay 1922**).

All this signifies that the body retains the anatomical and physiological substrates (i.e. electrical excitability) that mediate these movements, both neural and muscular, for at least several hours. Of course, this is not tantamount to restoration of awareness to the subject.

Enter the Guillotine. Since its widespread use at the height of the French Revolution (and until 1977, when the last such execution took place), some believed the heads were still aware for a time after the beheading. The only way to be certain would have been to revive the head and ask directly.

Early in the XIX century, Dr JC Legallois in France proposed to *"reanimate life after death"* by *"replacing""the natural circulation"*. In this case, a physician could *"resurrect a cadaver some time after its death"*. In particular, he envisioned a blood transfusion experiment, with references to similar experiments by Bichat and Magendie (**LeGallois 1812, 1830**).

In 1857 French neurologist Brown-Sequard cut the head off a dog and did what Legallois had written about. The injection **started 8 minutes after decapitation: 2-3 minutes later he noted movements of the eyes and facial muscles that appeared voluntarily directed** (see **Loye 1889**).

Starting in 1884, human heads were dispatched to the lab of Dr Jean Baptiste Vincent Laborde, where he would quickly bore holes in the skull and insert needles into the brain in an attempt to electrically trigger neural responses; he would also try to **resuscitate the heads with a supply of blood**. In one of these "patients" (Campi), 1hour 20 minutes had passed between decapitation and the start of the experiment. Generally, the lag was only a few minutes. In one, he ran current through the needles and the subject slowly opened one eye, along with twitches of the lips and jaw. In another, the head arrived to his lab 7 minutes after the beheading. He **injected oxygenated cow's blood and connected the arteries on the other side to those of a dog**. Muscles on the eyelids forehead and jaw could be made to contract and the jaw snapped forcefully. **Circulation was started 20 minutes after the execution**. No successful revivification ensued (but this remains the first known attempt at "resurrecting" the dead) (**Laborde 1884, 1885a,b**) (**NOTE 2**).

In sum.

Someone declared dead is best cast as someone who is not moving or breathing spontaneously nor showing any sign of relational activity. But the machine that props up (at least) movement is still there for some time. The question is thus: when does death, understood as a truly irreversible process, begin?

CHAPTER 2

SUPRAVITALITY

Thanatology, a branch of forensic medicine, investigates bodily changes that accompany the post-mortem period. This knowledge is utilized by law enforcement to establish the time of death of a cadaver and has broad legal consequences. One way to estimate time since death deals with so-called **supravital reactions**.

Spontaneous "supravital" activity has been reported in the XIX century after e.g. executions (references in **Madea 1994**). Opening and closing of the mouth and raising of the lower jaw, proning/supination/flexion of limbs have been witnessed up to several (7!) hours without stimulation (**Tidy 1881; see also Onimus 1880**). In 1872, Rosenthal thought it could be a useful instrument for death time determination and in 1960 Prokop confirmed it (see in **Madea 1994**).

What is "supravital" activity?

Once bodily tissues no longer receive oxygen and nutrients (a.k.a. ischemia), after a short **latency period (LP)** starts the **survival period (SP)** during which organs and tissues still show spontaneous activity. This is followed by the **resuscitation period**

(RP), after which the ability to recover wanes. In other words, these three periods encompass the maximal ischemic damage which is completely reversible structure and function-wise.

The **supravital period (SVP)** is defined as reactivity to excitation during ischemic conditions, irrespective of whether the damage is reversible (and thus includes LP, SP and RP) or not. So, the RP of skeletal muscle under normothermic conditions is 2-3 hours, but the SVP may extend in some cases up to 20 hours post-mortem (and even more for single myofibrils)! (Figure below; hpm: hours post-mortem) (**Madea 1994, 2002**).

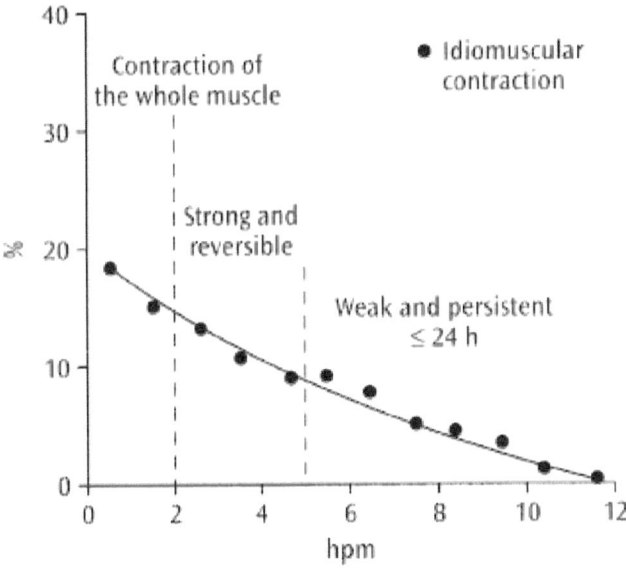

NB: The early (2-3 hours post-mortem) propagation of excitation of muscle after mechanical excitation is called the Zsako's phenomenon (1941).

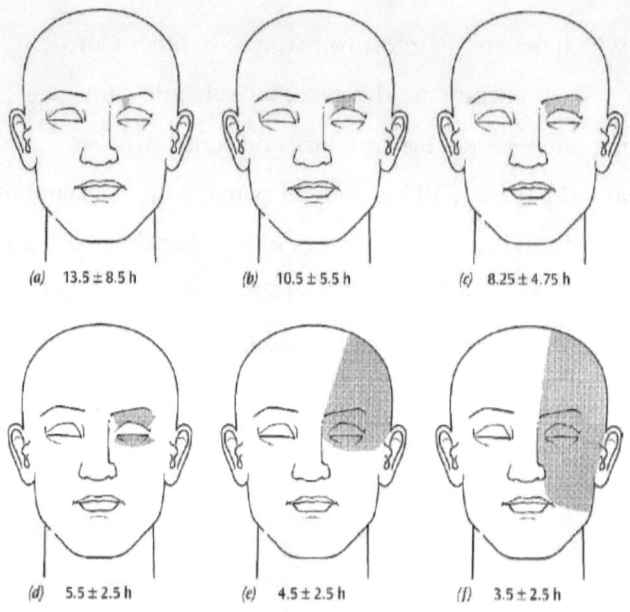

(a) 13.5 ± 8.5 h   (b) 10.5 ± 5.5 h   (c) 8.25 ± 4.75 h

(d) 5.5 ± 2.5 h   (e) 4.5 ± 2.5 h   (f) 3.5 ± 2.5 h

Degrees of reactivity (SVP) to post-mortem stimulation of the Orbicularis Oculi muscle by needle electrodes inserted in the nasal part of the upper lid (constant current, rectangular impulses, 10 ms/30 mA/50Hz) (Klein and Klein 1978, in Madea 1994)

The SVP is specific for each tissue. For the heart, these numbers are 3.5-4 minutes vs 100-120 minutes. Leukocyte motility ceases after a few hours, but phagocytosis is seen up to 68 hours post-mortem! Even supravital drug metabolism goes on for a considerable time. The iris can be made to contract for at least 1 hour post-mortem with drugs or electrical stimulation (**Madea 1994, 2002**).

We may conclude that –at least to some extent- the underlying anatomical processes that empower this "supravital"reactivity are **present for hours beyond the point of "irreversibility"**. The engine of supravital reactions is considered **vital metabolism** which after death runs down until exhaustion of substrates (e.g. glycogen) or until reaction-limiting changes of the milieu interieur set in: postmortem anerobic glycolysis runs at a high rate within the first 10 hours post-mortem, but slower afterwards and ceases at pH 6.3 (**Madea 1994, 2002**). ATP-asic activity is preserved in human post-mortem brains for some time (**Agafonov and Savulev 1976**).

In sum, it would seem that cessation of circulation and breathing is **not** followed by immediate loss of tissue "vitality" (**NOTE 3**). The question is whether the SVP, that may last up to many hours, may be leveraged somehow to extend the RP. In particular, it is time to consider the issue as it applies to the brain.

CHAPTER 3

ANIMAL SPIRITS

At the end of the XX century, two researchers (**Charpak and Audinat 1998**) conducted a grueling experiment, whereby they killed adult rats, some by decapitation. Dead animals or heads were left on a bench for 1 to 12 hours, the brain cooling naturally to room temperature (20–24°C) in about 25 min. Brain slices were cut at room temperature and left for at least 1 hr in a well containing a standard (20–24°C) oxygenated (95% O2y5% CO2) medium.

Their conclusions are worth repeating:

*"...during a permanent cardiac arrest, rodent brain tissue is "physiologically" preserved in situ in a particular **quiescent** state ...characterized by the absence of electrical activity and by **a critical period of 5–6 hr during which brain tissue can be reactivated upon [reperfusion and] restoration of a simple energy (glucose and oxygen) supply, [provided that brain temperature declines normally after cardiac arrest]**. In rat brain slices prepared 1–6 hr after cardiac arrest and maintained in vitro for several hours, cells with normal morphological features, intrinsic membrane properties, and spontaneous synaptic activity were recorded from various brain regions [neocortical, hippocampal, cerebellar, and thalamic]. In addition to functional membrane channels, these neurons expressed [undegraded] mRNA...and could synthesize proteins de novo. Slices prepared after longer delays did not recover. In a guinea pig isolated whole-brain preparation that was cannulated and perfused with **oxygenated saline** 1–2 hr after cardiac arrest, cell activity and functional long-range*

*synaptic connections could be restored **although the electroencephalogram [EEG] remained isoelectric**. Perfusion of the isolated brain with … picrotoxin…could **induce self-sustained temporal lobe epilepsy**…".*

In particular, cells from slices prepared after a post-mortem delay (PMD) of 1 hr and reoxygenated for 1 hr displayed a "normal, healthy" aspect. The average resting membrane potential of layer V pyramidal cells remained constant at PMDs of up to 9 hr. No cell could be recorded after 12 hours.

Recovery of function was seen after a 1-hour-long arterial reperfusion with an oxygenated medium heated to 27–30°C. **At least one major neuronal network could be reactivated.**

Brain tissue reoxygenation after ischemia is known to be associated with so-called **Reperfusion Injury** (RI). However, the drop in brain temperature occurring during cardiac arrest apparently prevented this cascade, which is highly temperature dependent: a 2°C drop of temperature (0.5°C/min) dramatically diminishes the damage during a 4-vessel occlusion.

Although rats are not humans, yet this study shows that **mammalian neuronal cells can survive "dormant" and be reactivated by appropriate means for several hours after cardiac arrest.** Possible delayed neuronal death after 12 hours at 37°C (the physiologic temperature of the human body) was not assessed.

What about larger mammals?

Experiments have been conducted on cats, dogs and monkeys involving similar global normothermic ischemia, including after decapitation.

CATS: In one experiment, cats were submitted to complete cerebral ischemia for 20 minutes to 2 hours by clamping the innominate and subclavian arteries and simultaneously lowering the systemic blood pressure. Neuronal function was assessed by recording the EEG and the anti- and orthodromic activation of the pyramidal tract. A full recovery of the pyramidal response and even of evoked EEG activity occurred after ischemia of more than 1 hour's duration! (**Hossman and Sato 1970**). In particular, under optimal conditions the D wave reappeared as early as 7 minutes after ischemia of 1 hour, the I wave after 25 minutes and the EEG after 45 minutes. Even after ischemia of 1.5 hours the I and D waves reappeared; the D wave did so transitorily after ischemia of 2 hours (**Hossmann and Sato 1971**). The 50 mosm blood-brain intra-ischemic osmolality gradient rapidly equilibrated upon recirculation in animals with signs of functional recovery, but remained elevated in those in which recovery was absent (**Hossman and Takagi 1976**).

DOGS: In a study (**Hinzen et al 1972**) mongrel dogs were euthanized and decapitated. After 30 to 60 minutes, the authors reperfused the brains and assessed them 1, 3 and 8 hours later. During recovery after ischemia of 30 minutes, cerebral cortical energy reserves were rapidly and completely restored to the normal range; incomplete recovery of the elctrocorticogram was observed **after 8 hours postischemic reperfusion**. After 60 minutes of complete ischemia, metabolic recovery was incomplete and only transient; no spontaneous electrocorticographic activity could be detected. However, strychnine solution topically applied to the cerebral cortices evoked electrical potentials during recovery after both 30 and 60 minutes ischemia.

Similarly, complete cerebral ischemia of 1 to 30 minutes duration was induced under normothermic conditions in completely isolated canine heads. The electrocorticogram returned following reperfusion from a donor dog's circulation. However, the longer the ischemia, the longer the latency of recovery, being of **11-12 hours after 30 minutes of complete ischemia** (**Hirsch et al 1975**).

MONKEYS: the cerebral blood flow (CBF) was completely interrupted for 1 hour in normothermic rhesus monkeys (macaca mulatta) and restarted at several time points after 45 min to 24 h in a series of studies (**Hossmann and Zimmermann 1974; Zimmermann and Hossman 1975; Kleihues et al 1975**). During ischemia, the electrocorticogram (EcoG) was suppressed within 15 seconds and the pyramidal response (PyR) within a few minutes.

However, in 11 out of 19 animals the PyR and — at survival times of more than 90 min — EcoG activity returned upon recirculation (in 8 it did not, presumably because of an impaired blood recirculation of the brain). Reduction in post-ischemic blood flow resulted from the combined effect of post-ischemic brain swelling with consequent increased intracranial pressure, microcirculatory disturbances, and post-ischemic hypotension. In one case the circulatory disturbance was restricted to circumscribed areas causing typical boundary zone lesions in the pallidum and parietal lobe. During 1 hour's ischemia, brain water did not change significantly, but the differences in the Na^+-K^+ ratio in white and gray matter were reduced. Blood recirculation of the brain caused a considerable increase in brain water content and a shift in the Na^+-K^+ ratio. Calculated brain swelling was maximal after 45 min when it reached 11.1% of the total brain volume in an animal with recovery and 12.2% in another one without recovery. Most relevantly, in animals with signs of functional recovery only, brain swelling rapidly diminished, followed by a more gradual normalization of brain electrolytes within 24 hours. Also, a partial replenishment of cellular energy sources (ATP, phosphocreatine) and a progressive normalization of cerebral lactate levels were observed. Glucose and pyruvate concentrations showed a transient increase over control values during the early stages of postischemic recirculation. During complete cerebral ischemia, both synthesis and catabolism of proteins were inhibited, but in recovering animals, these changes were reversible starting several hours after recirculation and achieving a normal profile 24 hours later.

In sum, global ischemia in cats, dogs and primates, as seen after complete interruption of blood flow to the brain, be it by cardiac arrest or vascular clamping, does not inevitably lead to "brain death" as, in several animals, neurons can be reactivated upon recirculation under normothermic conditions: they merely lie in a "**dormant**" state. However, some brain regions (CA1 subfield of the hippocampus, Purkinje cells in the cerebellum, small and medium-sized neurons of the striatum, and layers III/V/VI of the cortex) appear to be more vulnerable to ischemia and are thus in need of greater resuscitation efforts than elsewhere in the brain (**Hossmann 1985**). In particular, GABAergic neurons appear more resistant than excitatory ones.

PIGS: Pigs are interesting in light of the many similarities between our brains and theirs, at both cellular and network levels (e.g. **Simchick et al 2019; Jelsing et al 2006**). A group (**Vrselja et al 2019**) studied 32 pigs exsanguinated at the slaughterhouse and decapitated in their laboratory. The heads were flushed of residual blood with heparinized (2,800 UI in total), isotonic phosphate-buffered saline solution (20 °C). Brains were then extracted from the skulls: the epidural temperature following the craniectomy was 12–15 °C. **At 4 hours post-mortem,** brains were then selectively perfused **for 6 hours** with a special haemoglobin-based, acellular, anti-apoptotic and noncoagulative cytoprotective perfusate (see APPENDIX) in a custom-made pulsatile-perfusion device (BrainEx) and allowed to rewarm from 25 °C to 37 °C at a rate of 6 °C per hour, using a range of pressure parameters (50/35–80/65 mm Hg, 72 beats per minute). The cerebral perfusate flow was monitored and arterial pressure adjusted appropriately to maintain relatively constant cerebral flow. The heads were processed, stored, and transported on ice until the brain was extracted at room temperature. The main result of this study was that after 10 hours from death no flow could be restablished, but **before 10 hours microvasculature remained patent and maintained flow**. The entire brain was perfused with a **normal pattern** (controls did not). Arteriovenous gradients demonstrated consistent consumption of glucose and oxygen as the brains reached normothermia, with concurrent production of CO_2 and a physiological drop in pH.

In the end, treatment with the perfusate resulted in :
1-edema-free macro- and micro-structural preservation of the brain and integrity of both excitatory and inhibitory neurons and their synapses, including in vulnerable areas such as the hippocampus (all subregions), neocortex (prefrontal and motor), and cerebellum;

2- vascular and glial responsiveness to pharmacological (vasodilators) and immunogenic (inflammatory) interventions;

3-spontaneous synaptic activity and active Na+/K+ homeostasis;

4-active cerebral metabolism.

The electrocorticogram (EcoG) remained isoelectric, though. However, the perfusion time had been short (6 hours) and the perfusate contained neuronal inhibitory substances. Thus, just like other reviewed studies, no conclusion can be drawn as to whether much longer perfusion periods (up to days) might have led to reestablishment of neurologic function.

In conclusion

The mammalian brain is much more resilient to lack of oxygen and nutrients at normothermia than thought. A much longer window of opportunity for resuscitative intervention presents itself (several hours).

CHAPTER 4

BUCKING DEATH

Despite decades of study, the **only unequivocal sign of cell death** is morphological, i.e. **cell disintegration** (or phagocytosis). Data shows that ischemic cell death is characterized by a long delay between the insult and manifestation of major cell damage. This delay varies greatly, depending on the nature of the insult and the brain region being affected. In some cases, it is as long as **several days or even weeks,** whereas in others it is **a few hours or less (Lipton 1999)**. It is clear that, for any one region, the longer the insult, the shorter the delay.

As a rule of thumb, the time before the cell disintegrates is **between 12 hours and 4 days. The cytoplasm and cellular organelles such as the mitochondria are well maintained for the first 2 days (!) following ischemia (Kirino 1982, Pulsinelli et al 1982)**. In particular, **mitochondria remain functional for up to 10 hours post-mortem in human cerebral cortical tissue (Barksdale et al 2010)**. Afterwards, other changes set in and the cells are completely destroyed and disappear only on the 3–4th day! Physiologic and metabolic parameters are also maintained **for a few days, e.g. the membrane potential ($\approx$50 mV) and electrical excitation (Kirino 2000)**.

These observations apply to both animals and humans (**Lipton 1999, Love et al 2000**).

Kirino (**2000**) coined a name for this phenomenon - **delayed neuronal death** (DND); we will refer to it as **Resistance To Death** (RTD) (**Hossmann 1985**).

Cell death comes in several varieties, the two most common being necrosis and apoptosis (refer to e.g. **Lodish et al 2016, pp 1011-1022** for details; **NOTE 4**). Recent data shows that cells can survive transient apoptotic stimuli, even after executioner caspase activation, a process dubbed **anastasis** (**Tang et al 2012**). In particular, even in the presence of the classic apoptotic hallmarks (activation of caspase 3, cell shrinkage, and membrane blebbing), **removal of the apoptotic stimuli after a few hours** (e.g. by replacing the growth medium) **allows most cells to recover a relatively normal morphology**. Anastasis is an active process, rather than simply arrest of the apoptotic process. The early stage involves transcription of many transcription factors, stress response, re-entry into the cell cycle, and proliferation. Cells in the late stage undergo cytoskeletal rearrangement and morphological change and become more migratory (**Sun and Montell 2017**). This process likely applies to all kinds of cells.

Anastasis is not the only example of a reversible cell death process. Cells can recover from a variety of near-death experiences.

Resuscitation refers to the recovery from near death in cells undergoing necroptosis (**Gong et al 2017**). Even entosis, in which one cell swallows another alive, turns out to be reversible: the internalized cell can emerge to live again (**Overholtzer and Brugge 2008).**

In sum:

A cell in the process of dissolution can reacquire its normal morphology.

CHAPTER 5

BACK FROM THE DEAD

For the longest time, people believed that autoptic brain tissue is not suitable for experimentation because of the deleterious effects of the agonal state at death and postmortem delay on labile cellular constituents. Actually, studies going back to the 1970's confirmed successful neuronal culture from postmortem human tissue (e.g. **Iqbal and Tellez-Nagel 1972:** normal human brain specimens obtained **2-16 h post-mortem**). It was also observed how neurons in culture could survive longer than 60 minutes under anoxia, if the culture medium was low on Na+ and Ca++ (**Goldberg et al 1986**).

In the 1990's, data relevant to this book's thesis emerged, in particular evidence for survival of human brain neurons **up to 8 hours** (!) **after death** such that they still had the potential to recover their functions of energy metabolism and axonal transport (**Dai et al 1998**): biotinylated dextran amine, an axonal tracer, was transported in the hypothalamus over 1– 2 cm during the first 24 h after autopsy.

In a follow-up study (**Verwer et al 2002**) the authors removed the brain from cadavers 2–8 hours postmortem (mean: 4.2 hours). Tissue cultures of brain slices showed survival of viable neurons with normal morphology from both cortex (including the primary motor cortex, M1) and subcortical brain areas. Neurons from M1 were maintained in culture for 1 up to 78 days (Figure below)! Material from nearly two-thirds of the patients could be used for experiments lasting at least 3 weeks and about half of the cultures could be used for more than 30 days.

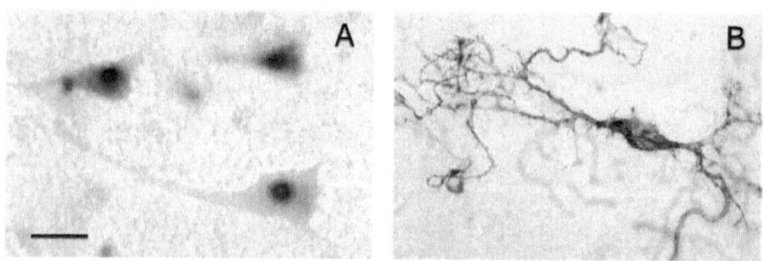

Vital human motor cortex pyramidal cells in culture; post-mortem interval: 5 hours; (From: Verwer et al. Life after death? Neurology 2002;1335)

Some populations of neurons were more resistant than others. For instance, layer II cells of the motor cortex and pyramidal cells of the Cornu Ammonis region of the hippocampus appeared to be relatively vulnerable, whereas large pyramidal cells in layers III and V of the motor cortex, hippocampal hilar cells, dentate gyrus granular cells, and cerebellar Purkinje cells were not. The transport of biotinylated dextran amine in their slice cultures appeared to be selective, with the tracer mainly found in axons and less frequently in apical dendrites, and only rarely in basal dendrites (**Verwer et al 2003**).

In sum:

Human brain cells appear to have an intrinsic capacity to resist death for many hours following cessation of vital functions.

This should not be surprising. Mature neurons, in light of their irreplaceability, come endowed with multiple – both pre- and post-mitochondrial- apoptotic brakes, making them markedly more resistant to diverse cellular insults and cell death than immature, developing neurons (**Kole et al 2013**). In particular, different cells have different thresholds for the lethal level of caspase 3 activity.

Further data supports the notion that **dormant neurons can be reawakened**.

*"The (human) brain is left in the skull during the postmortem interval and cells that have survived the agonal state and this postmortem interval presumably have reached a kind of **resting state** when they are finally manipulated and placed in the culture medium. The morphological features of neurons and their histological organization in postmortem tissue slices may remain intact for as long as **50 days** in vitro (DIV)... While the number of viable neurons and the respiratory chain enzyme activity (cytochrome oxidase IV) gradually decrease... viable neurons may still be detected at more distant time points. Addition of **pyruvate**, a metabolite that can be directly used by mitochondria, prolongs the activity of cytochrome oxidase. Cells in these slices respond to experimental manipulation . For instance,... when we co-cultured slices with rat embryonic neural stem cells, which were separated by a semi-permeable membrane, we found a higher number of viable neurons than without stem cells. This suggests that rat **embryonic neural stem cells secrete molecules that are beneficial to human neurons** in vitro. The presence of morphologically intact synapses and traceable axons suggests that communication between neurons in these slices might be functional. Indeed, spontaneous electrical activity can be recorded in human postmortem cortex slices in culture... Usually, recordings are made at ≈ 2 weeks in vitro, but in a single preparation, activity was detected at a single electrode after 63 DIV...the addition of **nerve growth factor, brain-derived neurotrophic factor (BDNF), and neurotrophin-3** appeared helpful to obtain improved activity. In this way, we recorded **spontaneous electrical activity** in postmortem slices at many electrodes simultaneously or in synchronized waves over groups of electrodes,and this was suppressed by the addition of ...tetrodotoxin to the medium..(which) showed that sodium channels were functionally active in vitro...field potential activity, sparse firing, regular spike firing, and burst firing patterns were produced by neurons in the areas of the electrodes. It should be noted that some electrodes can be inactive for a considerable time and then suddenly start to become active again"*.

These authors employed the **R16 medium** (see **APPENDIX**) at 35°C with 5% CO2; this was refreshed three times per week with 100 µL of R16 (**Wu et al 2008, Qi et al 2019**).

In other studies, at least some cortical neurons were successfully cultured in vitro under **normothermic conditions** up to 24 hours (with a decay over time) postmortem, with recovery of expected neuronal physiology, morphology and cytoskeletal markers within 5 days. The authors (**Viel et al 2001**) employed an optimized serum-free medium of their own invention: **Neurobasal/Hibernate A** (**Brewer and Price 1996**) with 2% B27 medium supplement (**Brewer et al 1993, Brewer and Price 1996**) and 0.5 mM glutamine. Hibernate A contains glucose, pyruvate, balanced salts, amino acids and vitamins; B27 contains five antioxidants (**vitamin E, vitamin E acetate, glutathione, catalase and superoxide dismutase)** and 15 other components (including **insulin, transferrin, selenium, putrescine, progesterone, corticosterone, T3, essential fatty acids and ethanolamine**). H-A/B27 is modified from Dulbecco's Modified Eagle's Medium (DMEM) with the addition of **vitamin B12** and **ZnSO4**, but without neurotoxic FeSO4 and glutamate. H-A/B27 has lower osmolarity than DMEM and lower cysteine and glutamine concentrations. Cells were incubated in this medium at 37°C in a humidified atmosphere of 5% CO2 and 9% O2 .

B27/Neurobasal/ FGF/DHEAS (**Brewer et al 2001**) achieved about 1% viable neurons in culture from postmortem human brains with a postmortem interval as short as 3 h. Here, cultures were initiated from three cases ranging in postmortem delay from 2.8 to 4 h. **Dehydroepiandrosterone** (DHEA-S) was as effective as

FGF in promoting survival of human cortical neurons. In two cases, the combined effects of DHEAS and FGF on survival were no better than either one alone. However, **at lower concentrations, DHEAS was synergistic for survival with FGF2, allowing one tenth of FGF2's usual dose.** Adding NT3 and EGF to FGF did **not** prove additive. Testosterone and estradiol similarly did not boost FGF/DHEAS effects. BDNF was not tested (see also **Blass et al 1994, Palmer et al 2001**).

In sum:

An appropriate medium can lead to morphological and functional recovery of human neurons (**NOTE 5**).

CHAPTER 6

TOWARDS AN ELIXIR OF LIFE

As previously mentioned, restoring circulation to bring oxygen and nutrients to the brain and body is not without risk, as it may bring about RI, characterized by neutrophil infiltration (inflammation), oxidative damage of capillaries and arterioles (with thrombus formation and more ischemia), edema and ultimately mitochondrial collapse (through opening of the mitochondrial permeability transition pores) and cell death. In rats it has been shown that **neurons often die a full 24 hours after blood flow returns**.

So, any resuscitation medium (RM) must act at multiple levels.

The culture studies reviewed in the previous chapter (see also **APPENDIX**) suggest several ingredients that must be integrated in a successful resuscitative medium. These include:

1-Glucose

2-Pyruvate

3-Salts

4-Amino Acids

5-Vitamins (B complex, C…)

6-ATP…

7-Antioxidants

8-Hormones (T3, insulin, corticosterone, DHEA-S…)

9-Growth Factors (FGF…).

The EBR-Fe perfusate will also include:

1-**Polymers**: These are one of the the mainstays of the EBR-FE perfusate. Several polymers act as membrane protectants and sealants, e.g. **polyethylene glycol** (or oxide; PEG/PEO) (reviewed in **Canavero 2013, Ren et al 2019**). Some PEGs are currently used as additives in organ preservation solutions prior to transplantation in order to limit the damage associated with cold ischemia reperfusion and the IV administration of PEGs of different molecular weights has emerged as a new therapeutic tool to protect liver grafts from IRI (**Pasut et al 2016**). **Poloxamers (a.k.a. pluronics)**, amphiphilic tri-block copolymers of poly[ethylene oxide] (PEO/PEG) and poly [propylene oxide] (PPO) in a PEOM–PPON–PEOM configuration (M and N denote the number of monomers in a block). The ratio of the number of hydrophilic PEO/PEG monomers to the number of lipophilic PPO monomers determines the hydrophilic/ lipophilic balance (HLB) of the copolymer, which in turn determines how the copolymer interacts with membranes. Poloxamers having lower HLBs (e.g., **P85**, HLB = 0.50, i.e. 50% hydrophilic, 15 PPO units) cross membranes and can transport drugs or DNA across plasma, while those with higher HLBs (e.g., **F-68**, HLB = 0.80, i.e. 80%

hydrophilic, 29 PPO units) insert into lipid bilayers and can restore the integrity of damaged membranes. **F-68 (F-68) (PEO/PEG76– PPO29–PEO/PEG76**), a.k.a. **poloxamer 188** administered 48 hours after oxygen–glucose deprivation (OGD) rescued neurons from death in a dose-dependent manner. After 60 minutes of OGD, a proportion of untreated neurons died within 1 hour, likely by necrosis, while the remainder of the death, which began at 6 h and progressed over 48 hour, was apoptotic. At its optimal concentration (30 µM), F-68 **rescued all neurons that would have died after the first hour after OGD** and restored intact neuronal function. **This level of rescue persisted when its administration was delayed 12-15 h after OGD (Shelat et al 2013, Wang et al 2017**). F68 inhibits lipid peroxidation and modulates early apoptotic responses, including reversing mitochondrial outer membrane permeabilization. However, F68's ability to rescue neurons from apoptosis 12–15 hours after OGD strongly suggests additional mechanisms (not NMDA antagonism). Ischemia triggers the synthesis of N-acyl ethanolamines (NAEs), endogenous lipids (e.g. NAE 16:0 or palmitoylethanolamine) which act as antiapoptotic and anti-inflammatory agents (**Garg et al 2010**). F68 may regulate this synthesis, given the dependence of apoptosis on mitochondrial lipids. Importantly, F-68 crosses the blood–brain barrier and appears safe for human use.

2-**Methylene Blue**: This atoxic drug can reroute electrons in the mitochondrial electron transfer chain directly from NADH to cytochrome c, increasing the activity of complex IV and effectively promoting mitochondrial activity, while mitigating oxidative stress. In addition, it is a powerful suppressant of neuroinflammation and more in general strongly inhibits neurodegeneration (reviewed in **Wiklund et al 2016, Tucker et al 2018**).

2-**Hormones**: Brain death invokes an acute deficiency in thyroid hormones (**triiodothyronine - T3 and thyroxine -T4**) which ultimately precipitates **mitochondrial failure**, including in cadaveric human donors prior to transplantation (reviewed in **Novitzky et al 2006; Cooper et al 2009**). However, level I studies that support use of T3/T4 as a form of salvage therapy of organs that would otherwise have been deemed unfit for transplantation do not exist and many level II studies, which do not endorse its use, are of poor quality (**Buchanan and Mehta 2018**). Actually, it is the **combination of T3, arginin vasopressin (a.k.a. ADH), insulin and cortisol or methylprednisolone** rather than the individual constituents, or any other combinations thereof, that produced the highest procurement rates (**Novitzky et al 2006; Cooper et al 2009**). Culture studies reviewed in previous chapters suggest incorporating these hormones in the perfusate.

Gasmediator approaches which have been studied for their neuroprotective effects include –among others- Hydrogen Sulfide (H2S), Hyperbaric Oxygen (3 Atm), and Molecular Hydrogen (references in **Ren et al 2016**). **Hydrogen Sulphide (H2S)** protects against RI, as shown in a pig study after 3 of hours of ischemia (**Villamaria et al 2014**). The protection is centered on the mitochondria. However, the suspended animation effect seen in rodents is not replicated in large mammals and in humans there is an indication that decreased O2 uptake is due to a toxic reduction in maximal aerobic capacity rather than to a regulatory effect on mitochondrial respiration (**Bhambani et al 1997**). Nonetheless, even in large species, data suggest that H2S supplementation during circulatory shock provides protective reduction rather than toxic inhibition of mitochondria-based cellular respiration. Pretreatment with H2S ameliorates RI (**Fries et al 2019**). Unfortunately, inhaled H2S may damage the airway mucosa and soluble salts may be toxic at peak. Only slow H2S releasing molecules should be considered.

On the other hand, **Molecular Hydrogen (H2)** looks promising: this has antioxidative, anti-inflammatory and antiapoptotic actions. Inhalation of H2 gas (1-4% or 66.7%) –also in combination with O2 or N2- improved cerebral infarction in multiple animal experiments. A randomized controlled study evaluated H2 on acute stroke with mild- to moderate-severity and a therapeutic time window of 6 to 24 hours (**Ono et al 2017**). The H2 group inhaled 3% H2 gas (1 hour twice a day). No significant adverse effects were seen with improvement in oxygen saturation and most importantly clinical outcome. H2 can also be dissolved in saline under pressure (0.4 Mpa) for 6 hours. Hydrogen rich saline protects mitochondria from destruction in the brain after reperfusion.

Several drugs have potential, but are in need of confirmatory experiments:

Phenothiazines: **Chlorpromazine** and **promethazine** independently produce certain parts of artificial hibernation (obligatory hibernators are naturally protected from RI) and were part of the "lytic cocktail" used as a neuroprotectant in the XX century. Chlorpromazine protects a number of tissues (liver, kidney, spinal cord and brain) from ischemia, especially when injected in separate doses. Promethazine provides notable attenuation of ischemia-induced neurotoxicity in vivo (reviewed in **Forreider et al 2017**). In a rat study, promethazine and chlorpromazine administered together 2 hours after ischemia onset conferred neuroprotection in severe stroke, most likely independent of drug-induced hypothermia (**Geng et al 2017**).

Phenothiazines have an anti-apoptotic effect by protecting mitochondria; they also decrease utilization of glucose. However, some of the animal studies used doses too high for clinical translation, although lower doses may still have some effect. In any case, given the "extreme" nature of the proposed undertaking, this may not turn out to be an insurmountable problem.

Valproic Acid (VA): VA has improved survival in animal models of otherwise lethal hemorrhagic shock and polytrauma at doses six times higher than the dose used in humans for the treatment of seizures (**Dekker et al 2018**). Fortunately the maximum tolerated human dose (140mg/kg) is equivalent to the dose observed to have clinical benefit in swine models (150 mg/Kg) (**Georgoff et al 2018**), without alterations of platelets or coagulation nor of EKG function. VA is anti-inflammatory. Although promoted as a pan-inhibitor of histone deacetylase isoforms (some involved in apoptosis and cell death in man) (**Williams et al 2019**), actually no significant changes in the acetylation status of histone and non-histone proteins were observed in healthy individuals (**Georgoff et al 2018**). In swines, administration of a single dose of VA (150 mg/kg) decreased neural apoptosis, inflammation, and degenerative changes, and promoted neural plasticity at 30 days after brain injury (**Chang et al 2019**).

Cyclosporine-A is claimed to protect mitochondria, especially in synapses, but a controlled study in man found no beneficial effects in acute ischemic stroke (IV bolus,2.0 mg/kg) (**Nighoghossian et al 2015**).

Metformin inhibits mitochondrial complex I and opening of the MTP pore and may be useful for RI.

Mesenchymal stromal cells can be derived from most tissues, but at present, bone marrow MSCs are the best characterized. MSCs have the ability to migrate to the site of injury and differentiate into various mesenchymal tissues to modulate tissue regeneration and repair . They also exert paracrine and endocrine properties secreting growth factors and cytokines that have mitogenic, antiapoptotic, anti-inflammatory and antifibrotic properties . They have been beneficial for acute repair of the kidney in various experimental models, improving renal function, reducing tubular injury and prolonging survival (**Pool et al 2019**). Although they can home in on damaged tissue, there remains difficulty in targeting the specific organ with systemic administration.

At this point, the astute reader may well ask whether any "resuscitative medium" as envisioned in this book stand a fighting chance to attain the stated goal, i.e. organ resuscitation (starting with the brain) or is merely academic gibberish. Happily, the answer is affirmatory.

Early in this century, Brasile's group developed a system (EMS, Breonics) for ex vivo normothermic perfusion of organs that experienced up to a few hours of warm ischemia (WI) and were thus no longer viable for transplantation (and intolerant of the hypothermic conditions presently utilized to preserve organs intended for transplantation).

This system was used on canine and bovine kidneys, rat hearts, human placenta and bovine limbs and finally human kidneys. The conclusion was clear-cut: organs which were previously thought to be unsuitable for transplantation due to excess periods of WI could be resuscitated and repaired! (**Brasile et al 2005 and references herein**). Repair mechanisms were upregulated: gene expression supporting new protein synthesis was observed under normo-(but not hypo-) thermic conditions. The presence of **exogenous growth factors** potentiating tyrosine kinase activation in the EMS perfusate was **essential** for this repair profile.

More in detail, kidneys removed <u>**2 hours** post-mortem</u> (i.e. 2 hours of WI) were resuscitated and repaired (transplant-grade) during <u>8 hours</u> of EMS perfusion. Most importantly, the period of EMS perfusion correlated with the degree of repair: **the longer the**

perfusion, the better the repair. So, 18 hours of EMS perfusion provided additional repair, with function achieved more than a week sooner than the kidneys perfused for 8 hours prior to reimplantation. Livers after 30 to 60 minutes of WI were perfused for about 4 hours at 34°C: these too were repaired.

In the presently discussed context, **repair of the cadaver's brain and organs may well require several days**, depending on the time elapsed between cardiac arrest and the deployment of the EBR "Frankenstein effect" protocol of our concern.

The EMS system is an ex vivo organ regeneration chamber, and thus of no use for our purposes. What interests us is the perfusate (see **APPENDIX**). The EMS perfusate is a warm (25°-37°C), (bicarbonate-)buffered, high osmolar, heparinized physiologic solution (any commercially available salt solution or cell culture medium, e.g., Hank's BSS, Earle's BSS, Ham's F12, DMEM, Iscove's, MEM, M199, RPMI 1640, RSM-210), which contains essential and non-essential amino acids, carbohydrates, metabolites, inorganic ions, serum proteins, lipids, hormones, nitrogen bases, vitamins, reducing agents and additional components for oxidative metabolism (many of these constituents are found in other similar solutions) and vasodilators. *It does not contain whole blood*, other than a blood component (e.g. red blood cells, serum or plasma): *lack of leukocytes and platelets helps limit RI*. This solution can refill the vascular and pericellular spaces. Importantly, warmth obviates cold-induced deleterious effects (edema, vasospasm, depletion of ATP stores, shutdown of ion pumps, glycolysis, and toxic free radical intermediates). Equally relevant, cellular repair of ischemic tissues with the perfusate prior to reestablishing blood flow appears to ameliorate RI. Inflammation is consequently forestalled.

Other solutions for normothermic perfusion are available and may be considered:
Lifor (*www.elimspringsbiotech.com/lifor/4590166925*) ,
AQIX-RS-I (*www.mayflowerbio.com/cpl/30/20*) and
Hemarina-M101
(*www.hemarina.com/index.php?rub=organ_preservation*)
after appropriate adaptation.

CHAPTER 7
EBR-FE DEPLOYED

Let's now consider a possible broad-brush scenario in which the EBR-FE protocol is deployed on a cadaver several hours after an irreversible cardiac arrest. Details will of course come only from field experimentation.

Let's turn again to the competitive athlete referred to in the preface. This individual suddenly drops to the ground unconscious. The medical team rushes in, feels the pulse, starts advanced CPR (inclusive of intubation and defibrillation). After 20, 30, 40 minutes -or even more, all efforts are stopped: the heart is still. In the usual scenario, this subject would be considered dead.

In the new scenario, the subject is rushed to the nearest hospital equipped for EBR-FE and attached to a custom-made perfusional machine (see **Marchioro et al 1963** for an early design). Notice that no hypothermia will be induced on-scene or at-hospital (see **NOTE 6**): temperature naturally reduces over time in cadavers.

The goals are clear:

1- interruption of the progression of damage;

2- restoration of metabolism and initiation of protein synthesis;

3- regeneration and repair.

The first act upon attachment to the perfusion machine is flushing away the clotted blood and ischemia-induced toxic substances from the cadaver's body at an appropriate systolic pressure. This is achieved with the EBR-FE perfusate that initial human experimentation will have perfected (**NOTE 7**). Notice that the first flush is with an **oxygen-free** EBR-FE perfusate to prevent an oxidative burst of free radicals that would injure the endothelium (RI). The fluid's temperature will match that of the cadaver at the moment of infusion.

After the flush is complete, an **oxygenated** EBR-FE perfusate at increasing temperatures (up to 37°C) is initiated. This may contain perfluorocarbons or other oxygen-carrying substitutes (with vasopressors and beta agonists added if necessary). The machine will comprise one or more perfusion paths for circulating the normothermic EBR-FE perfusate, a pulsatile pump, a heat exchanger, a gassing system for regulation of respiratory gases (O_2, CO_2) and pH (along with bicarbonate buffer) and other monitoring/sensing systems, all controlled via a computer. The perfusate is replenished continuously with new one for the entire length of the perfusion (24+ hours).

An adjunct arm to the EBR-FE protocol is **electrical stimulation**. Many non-mammalian vertebrates demonstrate profound functional recovery following extensive CNS injury but also in peripheral tissues, including limb regeneration. The regenerative potential of injured tissues is closely linked to the intensity of injury-induced direct current (DC) bioelectric fields (EFs) which increase upon injury and remain present for many hours to days (<10 mV/mm in intact tissues; the injury site becomes positive: anode). Enhancing endogenous EF can induce regeneration in those tissues of species where regeneration is normally not expressed. In particular, enhancing (likely up to 100x) these EF might trigger regeneration in mammals regardless of the time elapsed between injury and treatment (**Leppik et al 2015**). This is not far-fetched: adolescent humans can regenerate an amputated fingerprint fully from the distal phalanx including the nail, but only if the stump is not sutured and left open and hydrated. Currents of 30 µA/cm2 leave such wounds. This technology is expected to reactivate "dead" neurons (**Becker 1985**; **Baer and Colello 2016**), but is still in its infancy.

Much easier to deploy is direct stimulation of the brain, employing non-invasive brain stimulation (**Canavero 2009**), including transcranial low voltage pulsed EM fields and low field magnetic stimulation (1KHz-10 Mhz).

Repetitive anodal **transcranial direct current stimulation** (tDCS) (1mA, 30 minutes, resting interval of 1 hour) under normothermia improved neurological outcome and survival in a ventricular fibrillation/cardiac arrest rat model, if applied immediately (2'). TDCS was as effective as hypothermia administered as targeted temperature management (TTM) (**Dai et al 2019**). In the present context, tDCS cannot be deployed immediately, especially if the EBR-FE protocol is applied hours after cardiac arrest. However, it can be applied during the initial stages of reanimation.

Another useful adjunct is **external counterpulsation** which increases CBF (**Liu et al 2019**). It may also synergizes with non-invasive brain stimulation in post-stroke motor function recovery (**He et al 2016**) (**NOTE 8**).

CHAPTER 8
THE RISE OF WATER

What we have reviewed is enough to justify an EBR-FE trial by itself. Yet, on scrutiny, something appears to be missing.

Neuronal excitability, i.e. the ability of neurons to generate and propagate nerve impulses (Action Potentials-APs), is considered the sine qua non of brain communication (and awareness!). Yet, *"The supposition that we completely understand how neurons propagate signals, as suggested by most modern electrophysiology and neuroscience textbooks, is ... a gross misrepresentation of current scientific knowledge"* (Drukarch et al 2018).

The question thus arises:

Should we understand better *"how neurons propagate signals"*, could we improve our resuscitative protocol?

I will not review the textbook explanation of how impulses are generated, conducted and transmitted by neurons, i.e. the ionic Hodgkin-Huxley (HH) cable model (1952). I will start with what is wrong with this view.

As early as 1912, Wilke, from the University of Heidelberg in Germany, advanced the idea that mechanical impulses underlie the propagation of information in nerves whereas the electric oscillations accompany these mechanical impulses. Wilke compared the neuron to an elastic hose and concluded that if a hose is capable of propagating a mechanical stimulus at a nearly adiabatic speed, then the same should be possible for neurons. He observed that *"One of the most persistent phenomena which is yet to be explained is the excitability of nerves by mechanical stimuli* [···]. *If you observe the appearance of mechanical excitability and further note that a stimulus caused by touch propagates at a constant rate, then you cannot fail to recognize the similarity with an acoustic wave; I do not mean acoustic waves in the ordinary sense, but **pressure waves**, which are very peculiar to elastic bodies"* (**Wilke 1912**). Hill (**1912, 1950**) proved that axons heat locally during the initial rising phase of the AP and cool by an equal amount during the recovery phase. The heat released during the first phase of the AP is not dissipated by passive thermal conduction, but is actively reabsorbed in phase with the change in voltage during the second phase of the AP, with no release to the environment (i.e. adiabatic and reversible). The HH model cannot explain mechanical excitability of axons, and actually predicts that irreversible heat is produced and released to the environment.

Ever since, considerable evidence (reviewed in **Drukarch et al 2018** and references herein ; see also **Le Bihan 2007** and **Mueller**

and Tyler 2014, Pollack 2015) indicates that APs are accompanied by

1-**variations in axonal radius, pressure (mechanical displacement) and length**. A complex, highly specialized network of actin filaments and microtubules runs parallel to the axolemma and forms a dense polymer-gel matrix which is cross-linked by Ca^{++} ions and structured water. In this new formulation, during excitation, the influx of Na^+ ions and **water** molecules displaces Ca^{++} from the gel layer near the membrane, thereby disrupting Ca^{++} bridges between the negatively charged protein strands causing the matrix to loosen and **expand** due to an increase in the repulsive electrostatic interactions (**axonal swelling**). These changes activate mechanosensitive Na^+ channels. In addition, the influx of Ca^{++} ions causes subaxolemmal actin-myosin filaments to contract, thereby in its turn accelerating the propagating axoplasmic pressure pulse. Contrary to the HH model, cytoskeletal integrity and presence of Ca^{++} are mandatory for any AP to be generated.

2-**production and subsequent absorption of heat**, i.e. reversible heat transfer (up to 23 μ °C): most -but not all- of the heat generated during the nerve impulse is reabsorbed by the nerve. Heat is released during depolarization as Na^+ ions travel down their concentration and potential gradients and subsequently heat is absorbed during repolarization as K^+ ions leave the neuron traveling down their concentration and up their potential gradients. Heat can be generated by the irreversible conversion of mechanical energy as the membrane stretches in an almost isothermal regime (i.e. with a small net production of heat which is irreversibly lost). Otherwise, heat is released when the membrane is subjected to a propagating AP, with ensuing local compression and an accompanying fluid-to-gel transition and creation of a wave. The fluid-to-gel transition changes both the area and thickness of the membrane and, hence, its capacitance. Since the membrane is asymmetrically charged, these changes appear as a voltage pulse and lead to a capacitive current.

In sum, mechanical forces and thermodynamics play a key role in neuronal excitability and signaling. How can we harness this knowledge?

Enter:

WATER!

Water makes up 60% (40 L) of the weight of any one adult male (55% in females, who have more fat, and 78% in babies). The water content varies in various body parts: **brain** and heart are composed of **73% water**, the lungs 83%, the skin 64%, muscles and kidneys 79%, the bones 31%. Water constitutes two thirds of cell volume and **more than 99% of the cell molecules are water molecules!**

Yet, contemporary thought would let us believe that such an ubiquitous component plays only a passive role in health and disease. No textbook will mention water as an actor in any condition (let alone as a supposed approach to revive a brain dead individual.

According to current teaching, the cell is enveloped by a continuous phospho-lipid barrier called cell membrane: if the cell membrane is breached, the cell dies. Actually membranes are made up of 50-80% proteins rather than fat. Anyway. **Poking holes in cells does not lead to cell death!** Even cells cut in two do not die: the nucleated one goes on indefinitely while the other half survives 1-2 days. In other words: a membrane is truly there but not to contain freely diffusible substances or water.

According to Gerald Pollack (**Pollack 2001, 2013**) (and not only, as we saw), cell cytoplasm is actually a **gel** and like all gels can undergoes profound structural **phase-transitions**. How does this happen?

Proteins dominate the cytoplasm: their hydrophobic element lies in the protein's core leaving the hydrophilic elements superficial and exposed to the water. As a result, **protein surfaces order nearby water molecules into a "structured" state (interfacial or 4th phase or exclusion zone –EZ- water)** made of hundreds of thousands or even a million or more layers **and provide adsorptive sites for charged solutes**. Since most water molecules lie within one nanometer of some hydrophilic surface, cell water is mainly interfacial water: its layering stems directly from the dipolar nature of water. The resulting protein-ion-interfacial water matrix has a gel-like character, which explains a cell's freeze-resistance and its ability to remain intact even when demembranated. As a (important) corollary, if **the cell is a gel, even dried animals can rehydrate to life, just as dried polymers can rehydrate to function.** It is the gel-like nature of cells that explains resistance.

   In more detail. Lying just inside the cell membrane is a dense **polymer-gel matrix**, a.k.a the peripheral cytoskeleton (PC), which is 100 times thicker than the former. "Transmembrane" currents flow through both. The PC is composed of cross-linked actin filaments and microtubules. In neurons, filaments cluster at distinct foci, while enmeshed microtubules run axially just beneath the membrane. Both are present in high density and both are endowed with **high negative** surface charge. Thus **the PC is a continuous shell of negative charge that envelops the cell. Actin has a proclivity to structure water.**

   Ionic composition of neurons is thus easily explained: negatively charged structured cell water excludes ions. Exclusion is more pronounced for Na+ than for K+ because Na+'s hydration shell is larger and thus more difficult to accommodate in the structured water. Importantly, n**o energy is required for maintenance.** Ergo, ion partitioning is not the result of pumps and channels (as in the HH model), but depends on the ion's hydration shell. Since Na+

ions are "excluded", they cannot balance out the negative charge borne by intracellular proteins, particularly the highly negatively charged proteins of the PC. Consequently, the cell is **negative**. Poking holes in a cell does not affect its electrical potential since **this depends on the bulk properties of the cytoplasm**.

(by the way: mitochondria are not saved by inhibiting influx of water through MTP pores, as proven by the negative results of a trial of mitochondrial permeability transition pore (mPTP) opening inhibitor TRO40303: **Atar et al 2015**).

APs in turn depend on phase transitions of the cytoskeletal gel. This dovetails nicely with what we have seen in the first part of this chapter. In particular this new view can explain why even in the absence of Na+ and K+, APs still happen! Equally, it explains why without an intact cytoskeleton or Ca++, APs cannot occur!

In the Pollack model, Na+ ions flow into the PC and displace Ca++ (the primary cross-linker), this replacement loosens the network, enabling it to **adsorb water** and expand (gel deconsensation). As it expands, permeability is increased allowing for more Na+ entry, further Ca++ displacement, additional expansion etc...this drives the AP's rising phase which is positive. The expanding matrix stores elastic energy. However, the matrix cannot expand indefinitely. Elastic retraction makes closely apposed polymers reaccept Ca++ bridges and **water exits**, restoring both the volume and initial cell potential (gel condensation).

If we look at mitochondria, a cell's power generators, water in and around them is structured. Mitochondrial surface charge continuously replenished by ATP structures vicinal water and structured water in turn drives nearby proteins to their extended high potential energy state, promoting order. Thus, **the energy for cellular action arises ultimately from charge**. The charge on the mitochondrial surface orders vicinal water which drives proteins to their extended state; charge on the protein surface extends the protein which orders vicinal water. Either way the protein water matrix gains potential energy. This potential energy can be used during the phase transition. **The energy–supply mechanism of ATP comes from ordering of water and extensions of proteins**. Said differently: ATP's negative charge and the protein's negative charge act to induce protein extension, which is critical for energy transfer.

How do we leverage this knowledge?

Pollack's group showed that agents known to enhance biological function (nutraceuticals and pain-relieving drugs) result in EZ expansion (although at excessive doses they diminish it, perhaps through an amplified production of protons with ensuing invasion and dissolution of the EZ lattice), whereas biotoxic substances considerably diminish EZ size (**Sharma et al 2018**). They concluded that when EZ water is deficient, proteins lie outside their "normal" environment and can be expected to misfold, impairing cellular function and therefore health. Conversely, rebuilding of cellular EZ water in EZ-deficient situations ought to return health toward normal.

The same group (**Kundacina et al 2016**) showed that anesthetics (Lidocaine, Bupivacaine, Isoflurane) at an extremely low concentration expand the zone of interfacial water, while at higher concentrations diminish it in a concentration-dependent manner (all effects fully reversible). The involvement of interfacial water would explain how elevated atmospheric pressures antagonize the effects of both liquid and gaseous anesthetics (**Miller et al 1973**): elevated pressure does in fact significantly increase the size of the exclusion zone (**Ypma and Pollack 2015**).

Are there ways to expand the EZ zone other than some chemicals?

Yes. As we have seen, next to hydrophilic surfaces, water molecules organize into hexagonal honeycomb sheets arrays (i.e. a lattice) casting off **positive** hydronium ions - $H+$ in the process. These multi-layered, low-pH crystals exclude (ergo: EZ water) many substances (including water and protons) and are commonly **negative.** The result is a **battery.** However, the EZ lattice has irregularities and can thus suffer erosion by $H+$ ions (which act as free radicals): these interact with the $OH-$ units making up the EZ and give off water molecules, thereby loosening the EZ's hexameric structure and opening the lattice. The EZ battery will need to be recharged. This happens when the sun's photons and other radiant sources (infrared in primis) dissociate bulk water and separate the charge (OH- vs H+). Recharging is best achieved by Infrared Radiation -IR (esp. 3000 nm), but also visible light and Ultraviolet Radiation (UV), in that order of potency (acoustic energy can also do the job). IR is always present, radiating from everywhere including the earth itself, but we also harvest energy from the sun, as UV goes deep into the body.

In sum, **water is an energy converter.**

IF this view is correct, **manipulating water is essential to restoring life. During the EBR-FE perfusion, infrared (thermal) irradiation (IRI) of the "cadaver" will be added to restore the gel structure of cells and thus neuronal communication.**

IRI has many biological effects and medical applications. It comes in three "flavours": near, mid and far IR. Far IR (FIR) is popularly known as "biogenetic radiation" and "biogenetic rays". The body experiences FIR as a gentle radiant heat which can penetrate almost 4 cm beneath the skin. FIR energy is sufficient to exert rotational and vibrational modes of motion in bonds forming the molecules (including water molecules) as well as resonate with cellular frequencies. FIR emitting heat lamps and garments made up of filaments (fibers) impregnated with FIR emitting nanoparticles are commercially available. Despite many applications, including the treatment of ischemia, the exact mechanisms of action are not well defined (but easily fit Pollack's view). FIR can also alter the human microbiome, which is essential to health (**Vatansever and Hamblin 2012; Shui et al 2015; Liebert et al 2020**).

All this should not be especially surprising. For instance, it is widely known that sun exposure has strong effects on the risk of developing multiple sclerosis independently of vitamin D: this effect is unexplained by current neurology, but is easily justified by the present theory (**Tremlett et al 2018; Langer-Gould et al 2018; Magalhaes et al 2019**), as would also be the faster rate of healing of daytime (+60%) than night-time wounds.

CONCLUSION

At the end, it has become clear that many current assumptions regarding tissue tolerance to ischemia need to be (profoundly) revised. Too many lives are lost because of current nihilism. Resuscitating a "cadaver" within hours of death appears to be grounded in (neglected) science. Patients in the "permanent" vegetative state can equally benefit.

The normothermic EBR-FE protocol, once proven effective, may even be deployed by EMS, which calls for a portable, light-weight, device, that includes a reservoir for holding the perfusate, a pump, sensors, a computer and a power source. The perfusate can be instilled via cannulation of a main artery (e.g. femoral, carotid…) from premixed, premeasured, replaceable plastic canisters, for a single immediate use. One canister contains EBR perfusate 1 for initial flush while another contains the oxygenated perfusate. Once in the hospital, the entire protocol is deployed (**NOTE 9**).

As a corollary, current protocols to rapidly (within the hour) freeze just-deceased heads (and/or whole bodies) for future reanimation might actually turn out to be successful, provided the de-thawing process does not damage cellular bodies (**Best 2015, Canavero et al 2016**)

NOTES

NOTE 1: The EBR-FE protocol may also be be construed as an extension of current efforts aimed at harvesting organs from circulatory-determined death donors (DCD)- namely, hyper-fresh cadavers- and keeping them viable. In this context, 5 minutes elapse between asystole and harvesting. Subsequently, **normothermic** regional perfusion is initiated with portable extracorporeal membranous oxygenation (ECMO) devices to restore blood flow (**Mowlem E et al. Am J Transplant 2017;17(suppl 3): 2165-2172; Messer S et al. J Heart Lung Transplant. 2018; 37: 865-869**). Cadaveric donation of bone marrow has also been reported (**Blazar BR, et al Blood 1986; 67: 1655-1660; Kapelushnik J et al. Bone Marrow Transplant 1998; 21: 857-858; Machalinski B et al. Transplant proc 2003; 35; 3096-3100**).

NOTE 2- As far as awareness is concerned beheaded subjects-wise, Dr. Beaurieux carefully described the head of an executed prisoner (Henri Languille) (1905):

"Here, then, is what I was able to note immediately after the decapitation: the eyelids and lips of the guillotined man worked in irregularly rhythmic contractions for about five or six seconds...I waited for several seconds. The spasmodic movements ceased. [...] It was then that I called in a strong, sharp voice: "Languille!" I saw the eyelids slowly lift up, without any spasmodic contractions – I insist advisedly on this peculiarity – but with an even movement, quite distinct and normal, such as happens in everyday life, with people awakened or torn from their thoughts. Next Languille's eyes very definitely fixed themselves on mine and the pupils focused themselves. I was not, then, dealing with the sort of vague dull look without any expression, that can be observed any day in dying people to whom one speaks: I was dealing with undeniably living eyes which were looking at me. After several seconds, the eyelids closed again [...]. It was at that point that I called out again and, once more, without any spasm, slowly, the eyelids lifted and undeniably living eyes fixed themselves on mine with perhaps even more penetration than the first time. Then there was a further closing of the eyelids, but now less complete. I attempted the effect of a third call; there was no further movement – and the eyes took on the glazed look which they have in the dead".

In the XX century, a scientist (**Derr RF. Life Sciences 1991; 49: 1399–1402**) ascertained that the time required for the oxygen tension in decapitated rat brains to decline to a level at which the brain becomes unconscious was 2.7 sec. He thus concluded that

"assuming that decapitation is a powerful arousal stimulus and that the resulting EEG activation (low voltage, fast activity) indicates a conscious awareness of pain and distress, the maximum time the pain and distress could be perceived would be 2.7 sec. Hence, decapitation of rats per se may be considered humane"

However, others found that the EEG of the decapitated rat head revealed conscious suffering for more than 10 seconds, although this has been disputed (**Hobson RR. Neurotoxicol Teratol 1992;14: 253–257**).

A group of Dutch scientists decapitated old awake rats during EEG monitoring (**Van Rijn CM et al. PloS One 2011; 6: e16514, Zandt BJ et al. Plos One 2011; 6:e22127**). Following decapitation, the power in the 13–100 Hz frequency band decreased according to an exponential decay function to half the initial value within 4 seconds. After 30-180 seconds following decapitation, a high amplitude slow wave was observed which they named Wave of Death (WoD) and signaled in their view the border between life and death. They concluded that in 4 seconds after decapitation the animal is unconscious, unable to perceive stress and pain. This number tracks well with results of others (2.7 –6 seconds). In another study (**Borjigin J et al. PNAS USA 2013;110: 14432-7**) the authors performed continuous EEG in rats undergoing experimental cardiac arrest and identified a transient surge of synchronous γ oscillations that occurred within the first 30 s after cardiac arrest and preceded isoelectric EEG. γ oscillations during cardiac arrest were global and highly coherent; moreover, this frequency band exhibited a striking increase in anterior-posterior-directed connectivity and tight phase-coupling to both θ and α waves. High-frequency neurophysiological activity in the near-death state exceeded levels found during the conscious waking state. They also showed in rats that asphyxia activates a brainstorm, which accelerates premature death of the heart and the brain (**Li D et al. PNAS USA 2015; 112: E2073-82**).

What about humans? This WoD has been studied in a case series of seven patients who were neurologically intact before withdrawal of care due to extensive systemic critical illness **(Chawla LS et al. J Palliat Med. 2009; 12:1095-100)**. Bispectral index (BIS) monitoring (or SEDline) was carried out in all. Loss of blood pressure was followed by a decline in electrical activity followed by a transient spike in activity that approached levels normally associated with consciousness. This high-frequency spike in EEG activity had short duration and the activity then declined to a level of activity associated with burst suppression. These end-of-life electrical surges (ELES) have been subsequently documented in animal and human studies by other investigators. Some have proposed that patients should not be declared dead for purposes of organ donation prior to the occurrence of an ELES. If clinical practice were altered to await the presence of an ELES, there could be detrimental consequences to donated organs and their recipients. These same authors then assessed 35 patients of which 7 were clinically confirmed as brain dead. None of the brain-dead patients displayed an ELES. Thirteen of the 28 remaining patients (46.4%) exhibited an ELES, i.e. high frequency EEG signal. This means ELES are NOT universal. The timing of the ELES appears to be within 180–360 s of the complete loss of measurable blood pressure. In addition, for the subset of ELES that have been witnessed by one of the investigators, the patients were motionless and appeared unconscious despite neuromonitoring that was consistent with an increased level of consciousness. The raw EEG signal that occurs during an ELES is of a higher frequency than the waveform that preceded them. No seizure activity was seen.**(Chawla LS et al. Death Stud. 2017; 41:385-392).** The exact cause and significance of ELES remain unknown.

As a corollary, a bold American physician even tried to measure the weight of the soul **(MacDougall D. J Am Soc for Psych Res 1907; 237)**!

NOTE 3- Gross motor movement of the lower right limb of a corpse **two hours** after apparent death is on record (**Nokes LD, et al. Med Sci Law 1989; 29:265**). Very old reports found that spinal motoneurons are dead after 25 minutes, and peripheral nerves after 35 minutes. Clearly it cannot be so.

Anyway. One should not be put off by the appearance of the cadaver if the time elapsed between death and resuscitation is within 12 hours (or so). A cadaver at 8-12 hours displays a characteristic lividity (*Livor mortis*): this merely consists in the deposition of blood in different parts of the body due to the gravitational force. It has no relevance to our resuscitative efforts. *Rigor mortis* (below) from loss of ATP would recede during resuscitation. Hypothermia, coagulopathy and acidosis, the triad of death, are specifically reversed by EBR-FE.

Table 1
Time course of cadavric rigidity

Rigor phase	Mean with standard deviation(s)	Hours postmortem					Number of publications evaluated
		Limits of 95.5% probability (2 s)		Variations			
		Lower limit	Upper limit	Lower limit	Upper limit		
Delay period	3 ± 2	–	7	<1/2	7		26
Re-establishment possible	Up to 5	–	–	2	8		–
Complete rigidity	8 ± 1	6	10	2	20		28
Persistence	57 ± 14	29	85	24	96		27
Resolution	76 ± 32	12	140	24	192		27

Mean and standard deviation calculated from the literature data of 150 years (1811–1960) by Mallach 1964 [43] (Schleyer [44] slightly modified).

Although most tissues are characterized by a sharp shift in gene expression at **around 6 h after death**, there are remarkable differences between tissues regarding the transcriptional response to PMI (postmortem interval). Some tissues (e.g., muscle) exhibit an early response, with most genes that change expression doing so right after death. Another set of tissues show a more sustained response, with gene expression changes of similar magnitude occurring through all PMI intervals. Finally, another set of tissues show a peaked response, with most changes occurring between the intervals of 4-6 h and 6-15 h (**Ferreira PG, et al. Nature Comms 2018; 9: 490**). In particular, immediately following death (and **up to seven consecutive hours)** there is an increase in the expression of many genes, and a decrease in the expression of a few. The majority of the changes in gene expression, however, occur

between 7 and 14 h post-death, with stabilization between 14 and 24 hours.

The most immediate biochemical change that occurs postmortem is a fall in the concentration of oxygen due to absence of circulation, resulting in a switch to anaerobic metabolism with the absence of the citric acid cycle. Anerobic glycolysis results in the accumulation of lactic acid (and ensuing fibrinolysis: **Takeichi S et al. Am J Forensic Med Pathol 5: 223-227; 6: 25-29; 7: 35-38**) and an increase in the concentration of NADH. In man, pH changes from 7.0 to 5.5 by 20 hours post-mortem (6 by 24 hours) (**Sawyer WR et al. J Forensic Sci 33:1439-1444**), while lactate concentration in blood post-mortem increases 20-fold by 1 hour after death and 50-70 fold by 24 hours (**Jetter W. J Forensic Sci 1959; 4: 330-341).** Lactic acid also shows the steepest increase within the first 6-8 hours post-mortem in the cerebrospinal fluid (see **Madea 2002 in refs**). Formate (methanoic acid), a catabolic product of several amino acids, does not raise for the first 24 hours (**Viinamäki J et al. Forensic Sci Int 2011; 208: 42-46).** The concentration of ammonia in plasma increases after death with a rapid rise after 8 hours (**Schleyer F. Forensic Sci 1963; 2: 253-293**). See **Donaldson AE and Lamont IL. PLOS ONE 2013; 8: e82011** for further discussion.

It takes 48 hours for white cells to start to decompose after death (**Penttilä A and Laiho K. Forensic Sci Int 1981; 17: 121-132**). In rat muscles, cell shrinkage by apoptosis is detected within 1 hour postmortem and reaches 33% by 24 hours (**Becila S, et al. Eur Food Res Technol 2010; 231:485–493**). Importantly, skeletal muscle stem cells –but also blood stem and progenitor cells- adopt a completely reversible **dormant (or quiescent)** cell state within 24-48 hours post-mortem and retain regenerative capacity up to 17 days post-mortem (**Latil M et al. Nature Comms 2012 ; 3:903**); mitochondrial activity is reduced and promotes dormancy, without significant changes in expression of pro- and anti-apoptotic genes. The resistance to severe hypoxia observed in cadavers may be a general mechanism of all stem cells.

The heart can survive intact up to 4 hours after cardiac arrest.

Kidneys must be salvaged within 1-3 hours (but can be transitorily replaced by dialysis in the EFR-FE scenario). The lung is not dependent on blood perfusion for aerobic metabolism, but instead can use a mechanism of passive diffusion through the alveoli for oxygen delivery: in dogs, lungs retrieved 1 hour (but not 4 hours) after cardiac arrest are still viable. Even so, 23% of lung cells are still viable at 12 hours after death (if the animal is ventilated, this figure rises to 74%). Importantly, **ventilating the lung at 2-4 hours postmortem maintains normal ultrastructural morphology**. An agonal phase before death is especially punishing to lungs.

Overall, after cardiac arrest, the entire body is pretty much "alive" for many hours and more.

As a corollary, studies from the 1970's showed that about 60% of the brains in patients diagnosed as "brain dead" for 48 hours had no signs of necrosis at all.

NOTE 4: During intrinsic apoptosis, as induced by global brain ischemia, pores are formed in the OMM (outer mitochondrial membrane) in a process termed MOMP (mitochondrial outer membrane permeabilization) following production of apoptosis-inducing sphingomyelin metabolites. Similarly, peroxidation of cardiolipin in the inner mitochondrial membrane and its subsequent redistribution to the outer membrane are required for mitochondrial release of proapoptotic factors. Activation of the executioner caspases (3 and 7) occurs rapidly (20 mins).
This "suicide" process is initiated at one (or a few) discrete focus in the cell and then spreads via self-sustaining **apoptotic trigger waves** over large distances through the cytoplasm with speeds of **~30 micrometers per minute (Cheng XR and Ferrell JE Jr. Science 2018; 361, 607–612)**. The speed of these waves depends primarily upon the concentration of mitochondria (slower waves are possible in mitochondria-poor areas). Inhibition of executioner can slow, but not abolish these waves.
Whatever the cell death process of concern, i.e. necrosis or apoptosis, dying cells signal their status to the surrounding cells by translocation of phosphatidylserine phospholipids (PS) from the inner leaflet of the plasma membrane to the external leaflet.

NOTE 5: It is also the case that astroglia can be turned into neurons in vitro (**Zhang L et al. Cell Stem Cell 2015: 17, 735–747**). A N2 medium consisting of DMEM/F12, 10% FBS, penicillin/streptomycin, and 3.5mM glucose, supplemented with B27, 10 ng/ml EGF, and 10 ng/ml FGF-2 is utilized, with cells maintained at 37°C in humidified air with 5% CO_2. For reprogramming (MCM treatment), astrocytes are treated with TTNPB (0.5 mM), SB431542 (5 mM), LDN193189 (0.25 mM), and Tzv (0.5 mM) for 2 days. On Day 3, the culture medium is replaced with a different set of small molecules including CHIR99021 (1.5 mM), DAPT (5 mM), VPA (0.5 mM), and Tzv (0.5 mM). On Day 5, VPA is withdrawn by replacing the medium with medium containing only CHIR99021 (1.5 mM), DAPT (5 mM), and Tzv (0.5 mM). On Day 7, the medium is replaced again with medium containing SAG (0.1 mM), Purmo (0.1 mM) and Tzv (0.5 mM). On D9, the medium is completely replaced with neuronal differentiation medium (NDM), which included DMEM/F12 , 0.5% FBS, 3.5 mM glucose, penicillin/streptomycin, and N2 supplement. 200 ml NDM is added every week to keep the osmolarity constant. To promote synaptic maturation of converted neurons, **BDNF** (20 ng/ml), **IGF-1 (**10 ng/ml), and **NT3** (10 ng/ml) are added in NDM on Day 9 and are refreshed every 4 days until Day 30. This protocol may not be readily applicable in vivo (**Li H et al. Neuron. 2016 ;91:728-738**), but other protocols seem to work, e.g. dbcAMP, Forskolin, ISX9, CHIR99021, I-BET151 and Y-27632 (plus **BDNF** and **GDNF**) (**Ma Y et al. 2018 http://dx.doi.org/10.1101/305185**). The astute reader immediately understands how this fits into the EBR-FE protocol, should some damage be left after resuscitation.

An alternative would be using human brain organoids, that become vascularized after implantation (**Mansour AA et al. Nat Biotechnol 2018;36: 432–441**).

NOTE 6: The EBR-FE protocol does not include hypothermia (HT). The cadaver is already hypothermic and further hypothermia may prove detrimental. However, HT is a way to protect the brain and a few words should be spent here. HT is neuroprotective at multiple levels during ischemia/stroke/anoxia (far more than barbiturates; see also **Viel JJ et al. Brain Res 2004; 1009:219-22**). It inhibits free radical (ROS) production, caspase-3 (apoptosis) and mitochondrial dysfunction, calpains, inflammation, neuroexcitotoxicity, and vascular permeability. Since HT is not able to reduce Ca++ influx or inhibit the release of excitatory glutamate unless initiated immediately after the insult, it follows that inhibiting ion overload is not a necessary component of neuroprotective effects for latent phase cooling. HT is equally effective for RI.

HT is routinely used in surgery with prolonged hypoperfusion or hypoxia. Full neurological recovery from prolonged asystole (>1 hour) has been reported in humans exposed to accidental HT and submitted to prolonged resuscitation (e.g. 9 hours) (**Gilbert M et al. Lancet 2000; 355: 375-376; Mark E et al. Int J Emerg Med 2012; 5:7; Hilmo J et al. Resuscitation 2014; 85:1204-11**). Aspiration of cold water is believed to induce rapid protective cerebral HT without parallel decrease in core temperature, justifying higher survival rates in drowned patients compared to other causes of asphyxia even at similar core temperatures.

Rewarming by **extracorporeal circulation** is performed using standard cardio-pulmonary bypass techniques with either peripheral femoral or central cannulation. The ECLS-flow is set to match the venous drainage. **Extra-corporeal membrane oxygenation (ECMO)** may be used after rewarming.

In dogs and swine, rapid cooling to 10°C via intraraterial infusion of large amounts of ice-cold fluid with very large cannulas allows 1-3 (3 in dogs) hours of circulatory arrest, during which surgeons can repair the arteries: almost all animals survived neurologically intact, so much so that a trial has been launched (**Tisherman SA et al. J Trauma Acute Care Surg 2017; 83 803-809; see also Moffatt SE et al. J Royal Army Med Corps 2017; 164 140-141**). In this Emergency Preservation and Resuscitation (EPR) study, HT is initiated via an intra-aortic flush of a large volume of ice-cold saline solution at a rate of 2-5 L/min in patients with a loss of pulse <5 min prior to hospital arrival or on hospital premises. Rewarming occurs at 0.5°C/min and blood is transfused; electrolyte (especially hyperkalemia) and acid base imbalances are corrected. A flush solution containing O2 and 2.5% glucose allowed satisfactory recovery of neurological function after 3 hours of cardiac arrest in dogs (**Wu X et al. J Cereb Blood Flow Metab 2008;28:302-11**). For patients who remain comatose after cardiac arrest, temperature targeted management (TTM) at 33–36 °C for 24 hours (48 hours adds no further benefit, other than more complications) improves outcomes (**Nielsen N et al. NEJM 2013; 369: 2197-2206; Kirkegaard H et al. JAMA 2017; 318: 341-350**): timing of initiation, specific temperature targets, or duration of TTM are undefined.

Chemical induction of hibernation in small mammals has yet to be translated into its human equivalent (**Lee CC. Annu Rev Med 2008; 59: 177–86, Asfar P et al. Critical Care 2014; 18: 215**), but suggests that nonhibernators are fully capable of withstanding extreme hypometabolism. Parenthetically, mammals enter hibernation in an environment of constant darkness.

NOTE 7: Traditional fluid resuscitation with crystalloids is mostly supportive, and does not address the specific cellular dysfunction caused by shock and injury. Saline resuscitation, especially large quantities, comes with numerous deleterious effects, such as hemodilution, coagulopathy, brain edema, inflammation and further cell damage. Massive transfusions come with negative effects too. Current trauma care favors minimal use of crystalloids and early administration of blood products; plasma in particular changes the expression of genes involved in metabolism, platelet signaling, and inflammation. However, transfusion-associated acute lung injury and circulatory overload, allergic reactions, and transmission of infectious diseases are still possible.

On the other hand, **Lyophilized Plasma (LP)**, a freeze-dried plasma product developed in the 1930s, is logistically superior to FFP (it can be stored in ambient temperatures as a powder for as long as 30 years, and subsequently reconstituted and administered within minutes following rehydration with water) and retains its factor function much better than FFP. LP is approved for clinical use in Europe and has been used by NATO forces for many years with good results. LP can be integrated in EBR-FE.

NOTE 8: An interesting approach to tissue reanimation is Mechanical Tissue Resuscitation (MTR). In the case of the spinal cord, 50 mm Hg (MTR50) or 75 mm Hg (MTR75) subatmospheric pressure applied continuously for 5 days with a rigid, fenestrated poly-L-lactic acid/polyglycolic acid (PLLA/PGA) shell abutted on the laminectomy site interposed between the cord and a polyvinyl alcohol (PVA) foam vacuum dressing trimmed to the size of the surgical defect to prevent compression has proven beneficial. The evacuation tube is tunneled under the skin and exited distantly. The incision is sutured closed, and the site covered with an adhesive film dressing to ensure an airtight seal of the wound and the tube evacuation site. The evacuation tube is attached to a computerized vacuum pump (**Zheng ZL et al. Neurosurgery 2016 78: 868-876**). In a swine traumatic brain injury study, a delay in application of the vacuum to the site of injury of 3 hours provided the same results as immediate application. A 6-hour delay still resulted in significant, although lesser, results. The brain can also be treated (**Argenta LC et al. Neurosurgery. 2012;70: 1281-1295**). MTR increases blood flow, decreases edema, modulates cytokines and inhibits apoptosis.

NOTE 9: Among possible future refinements we may cite the use of blood products from young donors ("rejuvenation effect") – although clinical studies found no effect of younger age on outcome (**Amico F et al. Med Hypotheses 2019; 122: 141-146**) and of the kinetic isotope effect (deuterium-based heavy water: **Li X and Snyder MP. Bioessays 2016; 38: 1093–1101**).

APPENDIX

TABLE I

COMPOSITION OF THE SERUM-FREE, CHEMICALLY DEFINED NUTRIENT MEDIUM R-16

Medium R-16 differs from medium R-12 (Romijn et al., 1984) by the omission of L-glutamate and L-aspartate, the addition of D-(+)-mannose and $MnCl_2 \cdot 4H_2O$, and a lower concentration of sodium pyruvate and sodium phenol red. Mainly because of the relatively short half-life of some constituents and/or their instability in the complete mixture, these constituents are kept in special stock solutions at $4°C$ or minus $16°C$ and regularly renewed. A detailed description of the preparation of stock solutions and medium, and maximum storage times is available on request.

Ingredients	mg/liter	M	Ingredients	mg/liter	M
Albumin * ca.	2600.0	40.0×10^{-6}	Biotin (vit H) *	0.1	0.41×10^{-6}
Glucose	3443.0	19.1×10^{-3}	D-calcium pantothenate	2.75	5.77×10^{-6}
D-(+)-Galactose	15.0	8.3×10^{-5}	Folic acid	3.0	6.79×10^{-6}
D-(+)-Mannose	10.0	5.6×10^{-5}	i-Inositol	8.78	48.7×10^{-6}
Sodium pyruvate *	50.0	45.0×10^{-5}	Nicotinamide	2.71	22.2×10^{-6}
			Hypoxanthine	0.92	6.75×10^{-6}
L-Alanine	2.01	0.23×10^{-4}	Thymidine	0.162	0.67×10^{-6}
L-Arginine-HCl	104.12	4.94×10^{-4}	Retinol (vit A) *	0.1	0.35×10^{-6}
L-Asparagine · H_2O	3.38	0.23×10^{-4}	Retinyl acetate *	0.1	0.30×10^{-6}
L-Cysteine-HCl *	7.09	0.45×10^{-4}	Thiamin-HCl (vit B_1) *	2.77	8.21×10^{-6}
L-Cystine-Na_2	38.33	1.34×10^{-4}	Riboflavine (vit B_2)	0.28	0.74×10^{-6}
L-Glutamine *	25.0	1.71×10^{-4}	Pyridoxal-HCl (vit B_6)	2.72	13.4×10^{-6}
L-Glycine	21.94	2.92×10^{-4}	Vitamin B_{12} *	0.31	0.23×10^{-6}
L-Histidine-HCl · H_2O	33.07	1.58×10^{-4}	Ascorbic acid (vit C) *	100.0	580.0×10^{-6}
L-Isoleucine	71.63	5.46×10^{-4}	DL-α-Tocopherol (vit E) *	1.0	2.32×10^{-6}
L-Leucine	73.70	5.62×10^{-4}	DL-α-Tocopheryl acetate *	1.0	2.12×10^{-6}
L-Lysine-HCl	106.90	5.85×10^{-4}	Linoleic acid *	1.0	3.56×10^{-6}
L-Methionine	21.25	1.42×10^{-4}	Linolenic acid *	1.0	3.59×10^{-6}
L-Phenylalanine	45.67	2.76×10^{-4}	Thioctic acid *	0.045	0.22×10^{-6}
L-Proline	7.78	0.68×10^{-4}			
L-Serine	30.72	2.92×10^{-4}			
L-Threonine	66.94	5.62×10^{-4}	Progesterone *	0.0063	0.02×10^{-6}
L-Tryptophan	11.26	0.55×10^{-4}	Triiodothyronine (T3) *	0.002	0.003×10^{-6}
L-Tyrosine	49.82	2.75×10^{-4}	Corticosterone *	0.02	0.058×10^{-6}
L-Valine	65.82	5.62×10^{-4}	Insulin *	2.0	0.33×10^{-6}
Choline chloride	6.07	43.5×10^{-6}			
Ethanolamine *	1.0	16.4×10^{-6}	Sodium phenol red	5.0	
Glutathione (red) *	1.0	3.25×10^{-6}			
Putrescine	16.11	0.18×10^{-3}			
Transferrin *	10.0	0.13×10^{-6}			
L-Carnithine	2.0	12.4×10^{-6}			
$CaCl_2 \cdot 2H_2O$	188.74	1.28×10^{-3}			
$CuSO_4 \cdot 5H_2O$ *	0.0025	0.01×10^{-6}			
$Fe(NO_3)_3 \cdot 9H_2O$	0.068	0.17×10^{-6}			
$FeSO_4 \cdot 7H_2O$	0.19	0.68×10^{-6}			
KCl	320.34	4.29×10^{-3}			
$MgSO_4 \cdot 7H_2O$	168.27	0.68×10^{-3}			
NaCl	6030.0	103.0×10^{-3}			
$NaHCO_3$	2762.1	32.9×10^{-3}			
$NaH_2PO_4 \cdot 2H_2O$	95.38	0.61×10^{-3}			
Na_2HPO_4	31.95	0.23×10^{-3}			
$MnCl_2 \cdot 4H_2O$ *	0.001	0.005×10^{-6}			
$ZnSO_4 \cdot 7H_2O$	0.20	0.7×10^{-6}			
$Na_2SeO_3 \cdot 5H_2O$ *	0.0079	0.03×10^{-6}			

* From stock solutions

From : Romijn HJ, de Jong BM, Ruijter JM. A procedure for culturing rat neocortex explants in a serum-free nutrient medium. J Neurosci Methods. 1988;23:75-8

EMS solution (Brasile/Breonics)

Table 1. Ingredients used during ex vivo normothermic perfusion using the exsanguinous metabolic support (EMS) system.

Ingredient	Amount	Ingredient	Amount
DL- Alanine	0.12 g/l	Menadione (Na Bisulphate)	0.00003 g/l
L-Arginine HCl	0.14 g/l	Myo-Inositol	0.0001 g/l
DL-Aspartic acid	0.12 g/l	Niacinamide	0.00005 g/l
L-Cysteine HCl H$_2$O	0.00022 g/l	Nicotinic acid	0.00005 g/l
L-Cystine 2HCl	0.52 g/l	Para-Aminobenzoic acid	0.0001 g/l
DL-Glutamic acid	0.2672 g/l	D-Pantothenic acid Ca	0.00002 g/l
L-Glutamine	0.20 g/l	Polyoxyethylenesorbitan monoolate	0.04 g/l
Glycine	0.10 g/l	Pyridoxal HCl	0.00005 g/l
L-Histidine HCl H$_2$O	0.04376 g/l	Pyridoxine HCl	0.00005 g/l
L- Hydroxyproline	0.02 g/l	Retinol acetate	0.00028 g/l
DL-Isoleucine	0.08 g/l	Riboflavin	0.00002 g/l
DL-Leucine	0.24 g/l	Ribose	0.001 g/l
L-Lysine HCl	0.14 g/l	Thiamine HCl	0.00002 g/l
DL-Methionine	0.06 g/l	Thymine	0.0006 g/l
DL-Phenylalanine	0.10 g/l	Uracil	0.0006 g/l
L-Proline	0.08 g/l	Xanthine HCl	0.00069 g/l
DL-Serine	0.10 g/l	Calcium chloride 2H$_2$O	0.265 g/l
DL-Threonine	0.12 g/l	Ferric nitrate 9H$_2$O	0.00144 g/l
DL-Tryptophan	0.04 g/l	Magnesium sulphate (anhydrous)	1.2 g/l
L-Tyrosine 2Na	0.11532 g/l	Potassium chloride	0.40 g/l
DL-Valine	0.10 g/l	Sodium acetate (anhydrous)	0.10 g/l
Adenine hemisulphate	0.02 g/l	Sodium chloride	6.8 g/l
Adenosine triphosphate 2Na 2Na	0.002 g/l	Sodium phosphate monobasic (anh)	0.224 g/l
Adenylic acid	0.0004 g/l	D-Glucose	0.01 g/l
Alpha-tocopherol phosphate 2Na	0.00002 g/l	Insulin	0.01 g/l
Ascorbic acid	0.001 g/l	Bovine serum albumin	30 g/l
D-Biotin	0.00002 g/l	Sodium bicarbonate	4.4 g/l
Calciferol	0.0002 g/l	Pyruvate	0.22 g/l
Cholesterol	0.0024 g/l	Transferin	0.10 g/l
Choline chloride	0.001 g/l	Serum	10 ml
Deoxyribose	0.001 g/l	B-cyclodextrin	0.5 g/l
Folic acid	0.00002 g/l	Chondroitin sulphate B	0.004 g/l
Glutathione (reduced)	0.0001 g/l	Fibroblast growth factor	0.02 g/l
Guanine HCl	0.0006 g/l	Heparin	0.18 g/l
Hypoxanthine	0.0006 g/l		

Further possible EMS components:

VEGF	0.20	g/L
chemically modified hemaglobin* or	216	mg/L
perfluorochemical emulsion*	20%	(v/v)
Coenzyme A	0.010 g/L	
flavin adenine dinucleotide FAD	0.004 g/L	
β-nicotinamide adenine dinucleotide DPN	0.028 g/L	
thiamine pyrophosphate chloride Cocarboxylase	0.004 g/L	
P-nicotinamide adenine dinucleotide phosphate TPN	0.004 g/L	
2'deoxyadenosine	0.042 g/L	
2'deoxyguanosine	0.042 g/L	
2'deoxycytidine	0.042 g/L	
thymidine	0.042 g/L	
adenosine	0.042 g/L	
guanosine	0.042 g/L	
cytidine	0.042 g/L	
uridine	0.042 g/L	
ATP	0.002 g/L	
AMP	0.002 g/L	
UTP	0.004 g/L	
TSH		

PDGF, FGF1/2, IGF1/2, EGF,somatomedins, NGF, HBGF,ECGF, TGF

Cytokines (IL1…)

Urogastone

Colony stimulating factors

Erythropoietin

Petastarch, hetastarch

Linoleic acid, arachidonic acid, linolenic acid, eicosapentaenoic acid, docosahexaenoic acid, oils

Modified amino acids, such as citrulline, ornithine, homocysteine, homoserine, β-alanine, amino-caproic acid

Vasodilators : Adenosine, cyclohexyladenosine, verapamil flunarizine, nifedipine, SNX-11, chlorpromazine, and diltiazem. acetylcholine, dopamine, bradykinin, and arginine, prostacyclin (and analogs, e.g. carbacyclin) and Mg^{++}

Table 2. The components of the perfusate solution and supplements added during *ex vivo* normothermic perfusion.

Perfusate	
Compatible cross-matched blood or recipient blood depleted of leucocytes and platelets	1 unit
Ringer's solution (Baxter Healthcare, Thetford, UK)	200–400 ml
Mannitol 10% (Sigma-Aldrich)	20–25 ml
Dexamethasone 4 mg (Organon Laboratories, Cambridge, UK)	2 ml
Sodium bicarbonate 8.4% (Fresenius Kabi, Cheshire, UK) to normalize pH	10–40 ml
Heparin 1000 iu/ml (CP Pharmaceuticals, Wrexham, UK)	2–4 ml
Augmentin 1.2 g	10 ml
Supplements	
Prostacyclin 0.5 mg (Folan, Glaxo-Wellcome, Middlesex, UK)	4 ml/h
Glucose 5% (Baxter Healthcare)	7 ml/h
Nutriflex® infusion (B Braun, Sheffield, UK) with the following added;	20 ml/h
Insulin (Novo Nordisk, Denmark)	100 units
Sodium bicarbonate 8.4% (Fresenius Kabi, Cheshire, UK)	25 ml
Multivitamins (Cerenvit®; Baxter Healthcare)	5 ml
Ringer's solution to replace urine output ml for ml	

* hemoglobin, stabilized hemoglobin derivatives (made from hemolyzed human erythrocytes such as pyridoxylated hemoglobin), polyoxethylene conjugates (PHP), recombinant hemoglobin products, perfluorochemical (PFC) emulsions and/or perfluorochemical microbubbles, e.g. perflubron emulsion Alternatively, **red blood cells (RBC)** may be used as an oxygen carrier: **about 5 cc of RBC per 500 ml of perfusion solution (that is, about 1%) is an effective amount.** After 24 to 48 hours of perfusion, RBC were not cretinated. An amount of RBC in this range does not present the problem of mechanical damage to the organ associated with blood-based perfusates.

NB: nitric oxide donors or carbon monoxide in the form of soluble carbon monoxide-releasing molecules (CORMs) can also be entertained.

NB: other substances to consider for an EBR-FE perfusate: vitamin E , selenium, glutamate antagonists and dimethylsulfoxide (DMSO)

BEx Perfusate				
Components	M.W. (g/mole)	Concentration (mg/L)	Concentration (mM)	Volume (mL)
Gas-Exchange				
Hemopure ® (HBOC-250)	250k (average)	130k	0,52	750
Metabolic compounds				
D-(+)-Glucose	180	1255,86	6,977	N/A
Sodium Pyruvate	110	31,427	0,2857	N/A
Cytoprotective Agents				
Hexahydro-2-imino-1H-thieno[3,4-d]imidazole-4-pentanoic acid (2-Iminobiotin)	243	0,28	0,00115	N/A
5-(1H-Indol-3-ylmethyl)-3-methyl-2-thioxo-4-Imidazolidinone (Necrostatin-1)	259	0,14	0,000539	N/A
Disufenton sodium (NXY-059)	381	0,38	0,000996	N/A
Sodium 3-Hydroxybutyric Acid	126	40	0,000317	N/A
Glutathione Monoethyl Ester	335	1,7	0,00507	N/A
Minocycline	494	1,7	0,00344	N/A
Lamotrigine	256	1,14	0,00445	N/A
5-(2,6-Difluorophenoxy)-3-[[3-methyl-1-oxo-2-[(2-quinolinylcarbonyl)amino]butyl]amino]-4-oxo-pentanoic acid hydrate (QVD-Oph)	513	0,04	7,79E-05	N/A
Methylene Blue	320	0,19	0,000594	N/A
Antibiotics				
Ceftriaxione	661	76	0,114	N/A

Osmolarity: 310 mOsm, Oncotic Pressure 10 mmHg, Density 1.017 g/mL, Viscosity 1.05 cP

Components of the hemodiafiltration exchange solution.

Components	M.W. (g/mole)	Concentration (mg/L)	Concentration (mM)	Volume (mL)
Exchange Solution				
Amino Acids				
Glycine	75	8,57142857142857	0,114285714285714	N/A
L-Alanyl-Glutamine	217	246,2857062	1,13495717142857	N/A
L-Arginine hydrochloride	211	24,00000088	0,11374408	N/A
L-Cystine	313	13,7142854828571	0,043815608571429	N/A
L-Histidine hydrochloride-H2O	210	12	0,057142857142857	N/A
L-Isoleucine	131	29,9999993428571	0,229007628571429	N/A
L-Leucine	131	29,9999993428571	0,229007628571429	N/A
L-Lysine hydrochloride	183	41,7142853142857	0,227946914285714	N/A
L-Methionine	149	8,57142849142857	0,057526365714286	N/A
L-Phenylalanine	165	18,8571428571429	0,114285714285714	N/A
L-Serine	105	12	0,114285714285714	N/A
L-Threonine	119	27,14285756	0,22809124	N/A
L-Tryptophan	204	4,57142871428572	0,022408964285714	N/A
L-Tyrosine	181	20,5714277828571	0,113654297142857	N/A
L-Valine	117	26,8571427428571	0,229548228571429	N/A
Vitamins				
Choline chloride	140	1,14285716	0,008163265428571	N/A
D-Calcium pantothenate	477	1,14285711085714	0,002395926857143	N/A
Folic Acid	441	1,14285717	0,002591512857143	N/A
Niacinamide	122	1,14285706457143	0,009367680857143	N/A
Pyridoxine hydrochloride	206	1,14285715885714	0,005547850285714	N/A

Riboflavin	376	0,114285715657143	0,000303951371429	N/A
Thiamine hydrochloride	337	1,14285712342857	0,003391267428571	N/A
i-Inositol	180	2,05714285714286	0,011428571428572	N/A
Inorganic Salts				
Calcium Chloride	147	243,4285686	1,65597665714286	N/A
Ferric Nitrate	404	0,02857142944	7,07E-05	N/A
Magnesium Sulfate	246	57,1428550285714	0,232288028571429	N/A
Magnesium Chloride		0	0,571428571428571	N/A
Potassium Chloride	75	283,3325	3,77776666666667	N/A
Sodium Bicarbonate	84	2232	26,5714285714286	N/A
Sodium Chloride	58	5474,285688	94,384236	N/A
Sodium Phosphate monobasic	156	40,2857136685714	0,258241754285714	N/A

(From : Vrselja et al 2019)

Composition of Cold Storage Solutions for Organ Preservation

Ingredients	UW*	Celsior	HTK	IGL-1	Collins‡
Na+ (mmol/L)	25-30	100	15	120	10
K+ (mmol/L)	125-130	15	10	30	115
Mg2+ (mmol/L)	5	13	4	5	30
Ca2+ (mmol/L)	—	0.25	0.015	—	—
Chloride (mmol/L)	—	41.5	50	20	15
Phosphate (mmol/L)	25	—	—	25	47.5
Sulfate (mmol/L)	5	—	—	5	30
Bicarbonate (mmol/L)	—	—	—	—	10
Glucose (mmol/L)	—	—	—	—	140
Histidine (mmol/L)	—	30	198	—	—
Tryptophan (mmol/L)	—	—	2	—	—
Glutaminic acid (mmol/L)	—	20	—	—	—
α-Ketoglutarate (mmol/L)	—	—	1	—	—
Lactobionic acid (mmol/L)	100	80	—	100	—
Mannitol (g/L)	—	60	30	—	—
Hydroxyethyl starch (g/L)	50	—	—	—	—
Raffinose (mmol/L)	30	—	—	30	—
Adenosine (mmol/L)	5	—	—	5	—
Allopurinol (mmol/L)	1	—	—	1	—
Glutathione (mmol/L)	3	3	—	3	—
Osmolarity (mOsm/L)	320	320	310	320	320
pH	7.4	7.3	7.2	7.4	7.0
Viscosity (cp)§	5.70	1.15	1.80	1.28	N/A

HTK, Histidine-tryptophan-ketoglutarate; IGL-1, Institute George Lopez-1; UW, University of Wisconsin.*Additional ingredients are penicillin G, insulin, and dexamethasone.†Additional ingredient is **polyethylene glycol** (0.03 mmol/L).‡ Euro-Collins has similar composition but with a higher glucose concentration (195 mmol/L) and omission of magnesium sulfate.§ Viscosity data refer to a temperature of 4° C.

Steen's hyper-oncotic, cardioplegic solution

Table 3. The perfusion medium used for 24-hour heart preservation.

Na$^+$	136 mmol/L
K$^+$	23 mmol/L
Ca^{2+}	1.3 mmol/L
Mg^{2+}	8.0 mmol/L
Cl$^-$	142 mmol/L
HCO$_3^-$	25 mmol/L
PO$_4^{2-}$	1.3 mmol/L
D-Glucose	6.3 mmol/L
Albumin	75 g/L
Cocaine	6 pmol/L
Noradrenaline	6 pmol/L
Adrenaline	6 pmol/L
T3	3 pmol/L
T4	2 pmol/L
Cortisol	420 pmol/L
Insulin	8 U/L
Imipenen	20 mg/L
Erythrocytes (Hct)[a]	15%
96% O$_2$ + 5% CO$_2$[b]	0.2 L/min

[a]When all drugs and erythrocytes have been added and mixed and the PCO$_2$ has stabilized, pH is adjusted to 7.40 by means of sodium bicarbonate.
[b]Administered through the oxygenator.

REFERENCES

PREFACE

-Canavero S, Massa-Micon B, Cauda F, Montanaro E. Bifocal extradural cortical stimulation-induced recovery of consciousness in the permanent post-traumatic vegetative state.J Neurol. 2009;256:834-6

-Canavero S. Textbook of therapeutic cortical stimulation. New York: Nova Biomedical, 2009

-Canavero S. Halfway technology for the vegetative state. Arch Neurol. 2010; 67:777

-Canavero S. HEAVEN: The head anastomosis venture Project outline for the first human head transplantation with spinal linkage (GEMINI). Surg Neurol Int 2013;4 (Suppl 1):S335-42

-Canavero S. Head transplantation and the quest for immortality. Amazon Books, 2014a

-Canavero S. Immortal. Why consciousness is not in the brain. Amazon Books, 2014b

-Canavero S. Textbook of cortical brain stimulation. Warsaw: De Gruyter Open, 2014

-Canavero S, Ren X, Kim CY. HEAVEN: the Frankenstein effect. Surg Neurol Int. 2016; 7 (Suppl 24):S623-5

-Safar P. On the history of modern resuscitation. Crit. Care Med 1996; 24:: S3–11

CHAPTER 1

-Aldini J. An account of the late improvements in galvanism, with a series of curious and interesting experiments performed before the commissioners of the French National Institute, and repeated lately in the anatomical theatres of London, to which is added an appendix containing experiments on the body of a malefactor executed at Newgate, and dissertations on animal electricity, 1793 and 1794. London: Cuthell and Martin & J. Murray; 1803.

-Laborde JV. Recherches expérimentales sur la tete et le corps d'un supplicié (Campi).Rev Scientifique 1884, Juin 21, 777-786

-Laborde JV. L'excitabilité cérébrale après décapitation : nouvelle recherches physiologiques sur un supplicié (Gamahut). Rev Scientifique 1885a, Juillet, 107-112

-Laborde JV. L'excitabilité cérébrale après décapitation : nouvelle expériences sur deux supplicié : Gagny et Heurtevent. Rev Scientifique 1885b, Nov 28, 673-677

- Legallois, Jean C. Expériences sur le principe de la vie, notamment sur celui des mouvemens du coeur, et sur le siège de ce principe; suivies du Rapport fait à la première classe de l'Institut sur celles relatives aux mouvemens du coeur. Paris: Chez D'Hautel, 1812

-LeGallois JC. De la possibilite´ d'opérer une resurrection. In : Legallois, Jean C.1830. Oeuvres de César Legallois. 2 vols. Paris: Chez le Rouge, 1830, vol. 1, pp. 132-133.

-Loye P. Death by decapitation. Am J Med Sci 1889; 97: 387

-Mottelay PF. Bibliographical history of electricity and magnetism. London: C. Griffin and Co; 1922

CHAPTER 2

-Agafonov VA, Savulev IuI.[Electron-cytochemical study of ATP-ase activity in the brain after death]. Biull Eksp Biol Med.1976;82:1503-6.

-Madea B. Importance of supravitality in forensic medicine. Forensic Sci Int. 1994; 69: 221–241.

-Madea B. Post-mortem electrical excitability of skeletal muscle in case-work, In: Henssge C, Knight B, Krompecher T, Madea B, Nokes L, editors. The estimation of the time since death in the early post-mortem period. 2nd ed. London: Edward Arnold; 2002. p. 164–206 (see also: Henssge C, Madea B. Forensic Sci Int. 2004; 144:167–175)

- Onimus M. Modifications de le'excitabilite des nerfs et de muscles apres la mort. Journ de l'Unto et de la Physiol Norm et Pathol, 1880, 629 pp.

-Tidy CM. Legal Medicine. Part I. London: Smith-Elder, 1881

CHAPTER 3

-Charpak S, Audinat E. Cardiac arrest in rodents: Maximal duration compatible with a recovery of neuronal activity PNAS USA 1998; 95: 4748–4753

-Hinzen, DH, Müller U, Sobotka P et al. Metabolism and function of dog's brain recovering from longtime ischemia. Am J Physiol 1972; 223, 1158–1164

- Hirsch H., Oberdorster G, Zimmer R., Benner KU. & Lang R. The recovery of the electrocorticogram of normothermic canine brains after complete cerebral ischemia. Arch. Psychiatr. Nervenkr. 1975; 221, 171–179 (see also: Hirsch et al. Pflugers Arch Gesamte Physiol Menschen Tiere. 1957; 265:281-313; 314-27)

-Hossmann KA, Sato K. Recovery of neuronal function after prolonged cerebral ischemia. Science 168: 375-376, 1970

-Hossmann KA, Sato K. Effect of ischaemia on the function of the sensorimotor cortex in cat. Electroencephalogr. Clin. Neurophysiol. 1971; 30: 535–545

-Hossmann KA, Zimmermann V. Resuscitation of the monkey brain after 1 H complete ischemia. I. Physiological and morphological observations. Brain Research 1974; 81: 59-74

-Hossmann KA, Takagi S .Osmolality of brain in cerebral ischemia. Exp Neurol 1976; 51: 124-131

-Hossmann KA. Post-ischemic Resuscitation of the Brain: Selective vulnerability versus global resistance. Progr Brain Res 1985; 63: 3-17

-Jelsing J., Nielsen R, Olsen,AK. Et al. The postnatal development of neocortical neurons and glial cells in the Göttingen minipig and the domestic pig brain. J. Exp. Biol. 2006; 209,1454 –1462

-Kleihues P, Hossmann K-A, Pegg E, Kobayashi K . Resuscitation of the monkey brain after one hour complete ischemia. III. Indications of metabolic recovery. Brain Research 1975; 95: 61-73

-Simchick G, Shen A, Campbell B, et al. Pig Brains Have Homologous Resting State Networks with Human Brains. Brain Connectivity 2019; DOI: 10.1089/brain.2019.0673

-Vrselja Z, Daniele SG, John Silbereis, et al. Restoration of brain circulation and cellular functions hours post-mortem. Nature 2019; 568: 336-343

-Zimmermann V, Hossman KA. Resuscitation of the monkey brain after one hour's complete ischemia. II. Brain water and electrolytes. Brain Research 1975; 85: 1-11

CHAPTER 4

-Barksdale K.A, Perez-Costas E, Gandy JC et al. Mitochondrial viability in mouse and human post-mortem brain. FASEB J 2010; 24: 3590–3599
-Gong YN, Guy C, Olauson H, et al. ESCRT-III acts downstream of MLKL to regulate necroptotic cell death and its consequences. Cell. 2017; 169: 286–300
-Hossmann KA. Post-ischemic Resuscitation of the Brain: Selective vulnerability versus global resistance. Progr Brain Res 1985; 63: 3-17
-Kirino T. Delayed neuronal death in the gerbil hippocampus following ischemia. Brain Res 1982;239:57–69
-Kirino T. Delayed neuronal death. Neuropathology. 2000;20:S95–7
-Lipton P. Ischemic cell death in brain neurons. Physiol Rev. 1999; 79:1431–568
-Lodish HF, et al (Eds) Molecular Cell Biology. WH Freeman & Co, 2016
-Love S, Barber R, Wilcock GK. Neuronal death in brain infarcts in man. Neuropathol Appl Neurobiol. 2000; 26:55–66
-Overholtzer M, Brugge JS. The cell biology of cell-in-cell structures. Nat Rev Mol Cell Biol. 2008;9:796–809.
-Pulsinelli WA, Brierly JB, Plum F. Temporal profile of neuronal damage in a model of transient forebrain ischemia. Ann Neurol 1982; 11: 491–8
-Sun GP, Montell DJ. Q&A: Cellular near death experiences — what is anastasis? BMC Biology 2017; 15: 92
-Tang HL, Tang HM, Mak KH, et al. Cell survival, DNA damage, and oncogenic transformation after a transient and reversible apoptotic response. Mol Biol Cell. 2012; 23: 2240–52

CHAPTER 5

-Blass JP, Markesbery WR, Ko LW, et al. Presence of neuronal proteins in serially cultured cells from autopsy human brain. J Neurol Sci 1994; 121: 132–138
-Brewer GJ, Torricelli JR, Evege EK, Price PJ. Optimized survival of hippocampal neurons in B27-supplemented Neurobasal, a new serum-free medium combination. J Neurosi Res 1993; 35:567-76
-Brewer GJ, Price PJ. Viable cultured neurons in ambient carbon dioxide and hibernation storage for a month. Neuroreport. 1996;7:1509-12
-Brewer GJ, Espinosa J, McIlhaney R et al. Culture and regeneration of human neurons after brain surgery, J Neurosci Methods 2001; 107 : 15– 23
-Dai J, Swaab DF, Buijs RM. Recovery of axonal transport in "dead neurons" Lancet. 1998; 351: 499–500
-Goldberg WJ, Kadingo RM and Barrett JN. Effects of ischemia-like conditions on cultured neurons: protection by low Na+, low Ca2++solutions. J. Neurosci 1986; 6: 3144–3151
-Iqbal K and Tellez-Nagel I. Isolation of neurons and glial cells from normal and pathological human brains. Brain Res 1972; 45: 296–301

-Kole AJ, Annis RP, Deshmukh M. Mature neurons: equipped for survival. Cell death and disease 2013; 4 e689
-Palmer TD et al. Cell culture. Progenitor cells from human brain after death. Nature 2001; 411: 42–43
-Qi XR, Verwer RWH, Bao AM et al. Human Brain Slice Culture: A Useful Tool to Study Brain Disorders and Potential Therapeutic Compounds Neurosci. Bull. 2019, 35: 244–252
-Verwer RW, Hermens WT, Dijkhuizen PA, et al. Cells in human postmortem brain tissue slices remain alive for several weeks in culture. FASEB J 2002;16:54–60
-Verwer RWH, Baker RE, Boiten EFM et al. Post-mortem brain tissue cultures from elderly control subjects and patients with a neurodegenerative disease. Exp Gerontol 2003; 38: 167–172
-Viel JJ, McManus DQ, Cady C, Evans MS, and Brewer GJ. Temperature and Time Interval for Culture of Postmortem Neurons From Adult Rat Cortex . J Neurosci Res 2001; 64: 311–321
-Wu L, Sluiter AA , Guo HF et al. Neural stem cells improve neuronal survival in cultured postmortem brain tissue from aged and Alzheimer patients. J Cell Mol Med 2008; 12: 1611-1621

CHAPTER 6

-Bhambani Y, Burnham R , Snydmiller G, MacLean IJ. Effects of 10-ppm hydrogen sulfide inhalation in exercising men and women. Cardiovascular, metabolic, and biochemical responses. J Occup Environ Med 1997, 39:122–129
-Brasile L, Stubenitsky B, Haisch CE, Kon M, Kootstra G. Potential of repairing ischemically damaged kidneys ex vivo. Transplant Proc. 2005; 37: 375-6
-Buchanan IA, Mehta VA. Thyroid hormone resuscitation after brain death in potential organ donors: A primer for neurocritical care providers and narrative review of the literature Clin Neurol Neurosurg 2018; 165: 96–102
-Canavero S. HEAVEN: The head anastomosis venture Project outline for the first human head transplantation with spinal linkage (GEMINI). Surg Neurol Int 2013;4 (Suppl 1):S335-42
-Chang P, Williams AM, Bhatti UF, et al. Valproic Acid and Neural Apoptosis, Inflammation, and Degeneration 30 Days after Traumatic Brain Injury, Hemorrhagic Shock, and Polytrauma in a Swine Model. J Am Coll Surg 2019 (in press)
-Cooper DK, Novitzky D, Wicomb WN et al. A review of studies relating to thyroid hormone therapy in brain-dead organ donors, Front. Biosci. (Landmark Ed.) 2009; 14: 3750-3770
-Dekker SE, Nikolian VC, Sillesen M, et al Different resuscitation strategies and novel pharmacologic treatment with valproic acid in traumatic brain injury J Neuro Res. 2018;96:711–719
-Forreider B, Pozivilko D, Kawaji Q, Geng X, Ding Y. Hibernation-like neuroprotection in stroke by attenuating brain metabolic dysfunction. Progr Neurobiol 2017; 157: 174-187
-Fries CA, Lawson SD, Wang LC, et al.Composite Graft Pretreatment With Hydrogen Sulfide Delays the Onset of Acute Rejection. Ann Plast Surg. 2019 (in press)

-Garg P, Duncan RS, Kaja S, Koulen P. Intracellular mechanisms of N-acylethanolamine-mediated neuroprotection in a rat model of stroke. Neuroscience 2010; 166: 252-262

-Geng X, Li F, Yip J, et al. Neuroprotection by Chlorpromazine and Promethazine in Severe Transient and Permanent Ischemic Stroke. Mol Neurobiol 2017; 54: 8140-8150

-Georgoff PE, Nikolian VC, Bonham T, et al: Safety and Tolerability of Intravenous Valproic Acid in Healthy Subjects: A Phase I Dose-Escalation Trial. Clinical Pharmacokinetics 2018; 57:209-19

-Hill AV. The absence of temperature changes during the transmission of a nervous impulse. J Physiol 1912; 43:433-440

-Hill AV. The volume change resulting from stimulation of a giant nerve fibre. J Physiol 1950; 111: 3014-327

-Nighoghossian N, Berthezène Y, Mechtouff L,et al. Cyclosporine in acute ischemic stroke. Neurology. 2015; 84 : 2216-23

-Novitzky D, Cooper DK, Rosendale JD, Kauffman HM. Hormonal therapy of the brain-dead organ donor: experimental and clinical studies, Transplantation 2006; 82: 1396-1401

-Ono H, Nishijima Y, Ohta S, et al Hydrogen Gas Inhalation Treatment in Acute Cerebral Infarction: A Randomized Controlled Clinical Study on Safety and Neuroprotection. J Stroke Cerebrovasc Dis. 2017; 26:2587-2594

-Pasut G, Panisello A, Folch-Puy E, et al. Polyethylene glycols: An effective strategy for limiting liver ischemia reperfusion injury. World J Gastroenterol. 2016; 22:6501-8

-Pool M, Leuvenink H, Moers C. Reparative and regenerative effects of mesenchymal stromal cells – promising potential for kidney transplantation? Int J Mol Sci. 2019;20: E4614

-Ren X, Orlova EV, Maevsky EI, Bonicalzi V, Canavero S. Brain protection during cephalosomatic anastomosis. Surgery. 2016;160: 5-10

-Ren X, Kim CY, Canavero S. Bridging the gap: Spinal cord fusion as a treatment of chronic spinal cord injury.Surg Neurol Int. 2019; 10: 51

-Shelat PB, Plant LD, Wang JC, Lee E and Marks JD. The Membrane-Active Tri-Block Copolymer Pluronic F-68 Profoundly Rescues Rat Hippocampal Neurons from Oxygen–Glucose Deprivation-Induced Death through Early Inhibition of Apoptosis. J Neurosci 2013; 33: 12287–12299

-Tucker D, Lu Y, Zhang Q. From Mitochondrial Function to Neuroprotection-an Emerging Role for Methylene Blue. Mol Neurobiol 2018; 55: 5137-53

-Villamaria CY, Fries CA, Spencer JR, Roth M, Davis MR. Hydrogen sulfide mitigates reperfusion injury in a porcine model of vascularized composite autotransplantation. Ann Plast Surg. 2014;72:594-8

-Wang JC, Bindokas VP, Skinner M, Emrick T, Marks JD. Mitochondrial mechanisms of neuronal rescue by F-68, a hydrophilic Pluronic block co-polymer, following acute substrate deprivation. Neurochem Int 2017 ; 109: 126-140

-Wiklund L, Sharma A, Sharma HS. Neuroprotection by Methylene Blue in Cerebral Global Ischemic Injury, Induced Blood-Brain Barrier Disruption and Brain Pathology: A Review. CNS Neurol Disord Drug Targets 2016; 15: 1181-1187

-Williams AM, Dennahy IS, Bhatti UF et al. Histone Deacetylase Inhibitors: A Novel Strategy in Trauma and Sepsis. Shock 2019 (in press)

CHAPTER 7

-Baer ML, Colello RJ. Endogenous bioelectric fields: a putative regulator of wound repair and regeneration in the central nervous system. Neural Regen Res 2016; 11: 861-4

-Becker R, Selden J. The body electric. NY: morrow Publ. 1985

-Canavero S. Textbook of therapeutic cortical stimulation. New York: Nova Biomedical, 2009

-Dai CX, Chen G, Chen B, et al. Repetitive anodal transcranial direct current stimulation improves neurological outcome and survival in a ventricular fibrillation cardiac arrest rat model. Brain Stimulation 2019; 12: 659-667

-He W, Au-Yeung SY, Mak M, et al The potential synergism by combining external counterpulsation with intermittent theta burst stimulation in post-stroke motor function recovery. Med Hypotheses 2016; 93:140-2

-Leppik LP, Froemel D, Slavici A et al. Effects of electrical stimulation on rat limb regeneration, a new look at an old model. Sci Rep 2015; 5: 18353

-Liu JY, Xiong L, Stinear CM, et al. External counterpulsation enhances neuroplasticity to promote stroke recovery. J Neurol Neurosurg Psychiatry 2019;90: 361-363

-Marchioro TL, Huntley RT, Waddel WR, Starzl TE. Extracorporeal Perfusion for Obtaining Postmortem Homografts. Surgery 1963; 54: 900-911

CHAPTER 8

- Atar D, Arheden H, Berdeaux A, et al. Effect of intravenous TRO40303 as an adjunct to primary percutaneous coronary intervention for acute ST-elevation myocardial infarction: MITOCARE study results. Eur Heart J. 2015; 36: 112-9.

-Drukarch B, Holland HA, Velichkov M, et al. Thinking about the nerve impulse: A critical analysis of the electricity-centered conception of nerve excitability. Prog Neurobiol. 2018; 169:172-185

-Kundacina N, Shi M, Pollack GH . Effect of Local and General Anesthetics on Interfacial Water. PLoS ONE 2016; 11: e0152127

-Langer-Gould A, Lucas R, Xiang AH, Chen LH, Wu J, Gonzalez E, Haraszti S, Smith JB, Quach H, Barcellos LF. MS Sunshine Study: Sun Exposure But Not Vitamin D Is Associated with Multiple Sclerosis Risk in Blacks and Hispanics.Nutrients. 2018;10: E268.

-Le Bihan D. The 'wet mind': water and functional neuroimaging. Phys Med Biol. 2007; 52:R57-90

-Liebert A, Bicknell B, Johnstone DM, et al- "Photobiomics": Can Light, Including Photobiomodulation, Alter the Microbiome? Photobiomodul Photomed Laser Surg 2020 (in press)

-Magalhaes S, Pugliatti M, Riise T, et al. Shedding light on the link between early life sun exposure and risk of multiple sclerosis: results from the EnvIMS Study. Int J Epidemiol 2019 (in press)

-Miller KW, Paton WDM, Smith RA, Smith EB. The pressure reversal of general anesthesia and the critical volume hypothesis. Molecular Pharmacology 1973 ; 9: 131-143

-Mueller JK, Tyler WJ. A quantitative overview of biophysical forces impinging on neural function. Phys Biol 2014;11:051001
-Pollack G. Cells, Gels and the Engines of Life. Seattle: Ebner & Sons Publ. 2001
-Pollack G. The Fourth Phase of Water: Beyond Solid, Liquid, and Vapor. Seattle: Ebner & Sons Publ. 2013
-Pollack GH. Cell electrical properties: reconsidering the origin of the electrical potential. Cell Biol Int. 2015;39(3):237-342.
-Sharma A , Adams C, Cashdollar BD et al. Effect of Health-Promoting Agents on Exclusion-Zone Size. Dose-Response: 2018: 1-8
-Shui S, Wang X, Chiang JY, Zheng L. Far-infrared therapy for cardiovascular, autoimmune, and other chronic health problems: A systematic review. Exp Biol Med (Maywood) 2015; 240:1257-65
-Tremlett H, Zhu F, Ascherio A, Munger KL. Sun exposure over the life course and associations with multiple sclerosis. Neurology. 2018;90:e1191-e1199.
-Vatansever F, Hamblin MR. Far infrared radiation (FIR): its biological effects and medical applications. Photonics Lasers Med. 2012; 4: 255–266
-Ypma RE, Pollack GH. Effect of hyperbaric oxygen conditions on the ordering of interfacial water. UHM 2015; 42: 257–264
-Wilke E. Das Problem der Reizleitung im Nerven vom Standpunkte der Wellenlehre aus betrachtet. Pflug. Arch. Gesamte Physiol. Menschen Tiere 1912; 144: 35-38

CONCLUSION

-Best BP. Cryoprotectant toxicity: Facts, issues, and questions. Rejuvenation Res. 2015; 18:1–15
-Canavero S, Ren X, Kim CY. HEAVEN: the Frankenstein effect. Surg Neurol Int. 2016; 7 (Suppl 24):S623-5